AN ATLAS OF
COMPLETE DENTURE PROSTHESIS

An Atlas of Complete Denture Prosthesis

Employing Biologic and Simplified Gnathologic Principles

JACK M. BUCHMAN

D.D.S., F.I.C.D., F.A.G.D.

Consultant in Prosthetics
New York Polyclinic Medical School and Hospital

J. B. LIPPINCOTT COMPANY

Philadelphia · Toronto

Distributed in Great Britain by
Blackwell Scientific Publications
Oxford and Edinburgh

Library of Congress Catalog Number 76-653711

Printed in the United States of America

1 3 5 4 2

This book is dedicated
to my very good friends
Dr. Leo McCallum
and
Dr. Ajax Menekratis

The two chapters on gnathology are especially dedicated to
Dr. Peter K. Thomas,
my friend and adviser, who has done more for gnathology and
perhaps for dentistry than any man I know.

Preface

There are many textbooks on complete dentures. Why another one? In order to answer this question I must review my own experiences in denture construction.

My introduction to subject 35 years ago was similar to that of most dentists—as a fundamental technic learned in dental school. Once in private practice, however, I soon realized that there were almost as many different technics for complete denture construction as there were dental schools. And, furthermore, no one technic solved all of the clinical problems all of the time. After many frustrating years of less than total success in denture construction and, in my estimation, after all too many failures, I recognized that there were underlying physiologic and mechanical aspects of the technology involved in prosthetics construction that I did not know enough about.

Why were the ridges "melting" away?

Why did so many patients experience discomfort in eating and swallowing?

What caused the lower jaw to protrude even after the denture appeared to be in excellent occlusion?

I resolved to learn as much as possible about physiologic and mechanical processes in order to answer these questions.

Many years of inquiry and of study, and denture construction by almost every technic known, have made it graphically clear to me that the restoration of function and aesthetics for the edentulous pa-tient, and the fashioning of a substitute for the skeletal scaffolding around which muscle function occurs, are no easy tasks. I have found edentulous ridges ranging from the high and tortuous to the flat and inverted. I have found, too, patients with any of these problems, singly or in combination, who would tolerate and accept unsatisfactory dentures, while others could detect the tiniest occlusal discrepancy or surface roughness and proclaim the fact loudly and long. There are patients who will accept enthusiastically an arrangement of teeth which is esthetically inferior, and, at the opposite extreme, there are those who demand a standard of esthetics and function that can exhaust your patience and empathy. It has become eminently clear that successful denture construction carries with it more than the satisfaction of the physiologic and mechanical requirements associated with oral tissues. In denture construction we must never forget that we are working with human beings who have their fears, their strengths and weaknesses, and their sensitivities. Developing the patient's complete understanding *before* denture construction begins is of paramount importance. Indeed, I have found that patient cooperation can mean the difference between success and failure.

This book deals in a detailed yet concise manner with the construction of the complete denture in all its phases and variations—from those needed by the patient who has never had them before to those involving that tough, hard-to-fit, ulcer-producing flat lower ridge. Some of the technics explained here may seem troublesome, time consuming and difficult, but we agree, I think, that our patients, though some are difficult to treat, deserve our best and that our responsibility to them requires that we perfect our technics and increase our abilities.

Unfamiliar procedures often seem complicated, but as one becomes familiar with the underlying concepts, and as one practices, they soon become routine. When implementing *some* of the procedures I describe in these pages, you will need to follow every detail. In others, you can leave out certain steps at your own discretion. In all cases, however, give your patient the benefit of the most accurate scientific and biologic knowledge, the most advanced technical achievement and the best clinical skill.

With humility and with a deep feeling of gratitude to many of my teachers, it is my conviction that this book offers a complete denture technic, which, when carefully executed, will satisfy the requirements of aesthetics, function and comfort of the most demanding dentists and patients.

ACKNOWLEDGMENTS

It would be presumptuous for any dentist to say in our time that he had *independently* developed an original technic. Sometimes we become under-excited about a small innovation or a technic we have seemingly invented—until we discover buried in the literature virtually the same technic. Certainly materials have changed, as have technics, but each of us stands on the shoulders of someone who came before us.

I have spent many years in post graduate training. I have culled the literature. I have made some changes to existing technics. But what I believe I have done essentially is distill and combine, extending the ideas of many men besides myself.

I owe much to numerous teachers for their unselfish guidance and instruction. It was the late Dr. Russell W. Tench who first opened my mind to the ramifications of muscle function in swallowing and thus enabled me to develop a specialized concept of its use in the attainment of correct vertical and a tentative centric relation. I was fortunate to have been able to spend a great deal of time with the late Dr. Claude J. Stansbury, who taught me much about the central bearing and its principles. I am deeply indebted also to Drs. Carl Boucher, Joseph Landa, Irving Hardy, Richard Kingery, Sidney Silverman, Meyer Silverman, Muller M. De Van, Victor Steffel and Vincent Trapozzano. These teachers, by imparting their knowledge, helped me greatly.

I wish to express my gratitude for the teaching and kindness of Drs. Peter K. Thomas, Nils Guichet, Robert J. Pinkerton, Charles E. Stuart, Frank Celenza, Harold Gelb, and Harold Levine, Mr. Phil Larson, Mr. Clark Smith, the Detroit Study Club and the late Mr. Bernard Scullin and Drs. Thomas Shanahan, S.S. Jaffe, Victor Jaffe, M. Swenson and Dayton Dunbar Campbell. I also wish to extend special gratitude to my very dear friend, Dr. Nathan Allen Shore, whose continuing encouragement was a major factor in my writing.

My deepest appreciation to Mr. Tom Ito, my technician, whose outstanding skills and invaluable help cannot be described here, and to Miss Essie Mae Byrd, my devoted assistant, whose patience and talent have contributed so much.

It is my great pleasure to extend love and thanks to my only brother, Dr. Michael Buchman, an extraordinarily gifted dentist, whose keen mind and gentle disposition have helped so much. It was through his research and expert knowledge of the hinge axis that inspired me to development of the technic of denture construction I practice now.

. . . And to Evelyn, my wife, for the understanding and support she alone could provide, and so unstintingly did— an admiration I have expressed only inadequately before setting down these words.

Jack M. Buchman

Contents

AN ATLAS OF
COMPLETE DENTURE PROSTHESIS

1

Consultation with the Patient and Evaluation of Denture Problems

No case should be started until the dentist has had a thorough consultation with the patient and has fully evaluated his denture problems. If the patient is married, this consultation and evaluation should always take place with both husband and wife present. It has been the experience of the author that if the spouse is not present when the treatment program and fee schedule are discussed, the opportunity to benefit the patient through proper therapy is jeopardized because of the subsequent negative reaction of the spouse when the patient returns home. When the husband and the wife are together at the consultation and evaluation sessions, and when the practitioner has a chance to explain to both the scope of the undertaking and the problems involved, their reaction is more often positive.

The author usually takes two appointments for this consultation and evaluation, and the patient is informed that this procedure is a *must* before denture construction can be undertaken. The point should be made that denture construction is a painstaking effort requiring highly specialized knowledge and skill so that the final result will be specific for him alone; and he is made aware of the extent to which thorough preparation insures later health and comfort. In most cases, especially where the patient has had trouble with previous dentures, he will demonstrate no reluctance to pay a reasonable fee for such preliminary sessions.

During the first appointment, whether or not the patient is already wearing dentures, the procedures on the following pages are accomplished.

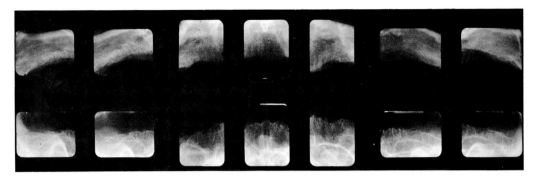

Fig. 1-1

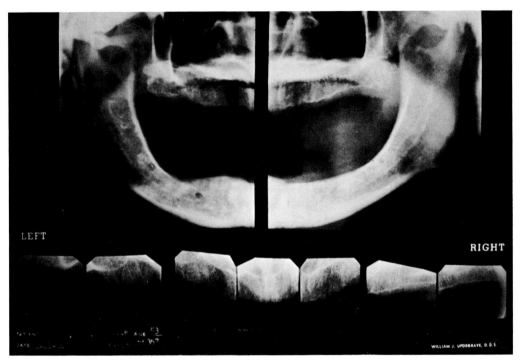

Fig. 1-2

1. A full series of X-rays of the mouth is taken, including a Panorex film if the necessary equipment is available (Figs. 1-1 and 1-2).

2. Accurate alginate impressions of the mouth are taken for study casts.

3. The fiber attachments of the internal and external pterygoid muscles are palpated for muscle spasms.[1] Checking for spasms, although rarely done in common

[1] Described in Chapter 6.

practice, is more than just a desirable step in the construction of dentures that are to be comfortable and well functioning—it is imperative. *If spasms are present and are not eliminated before the recording of vertical and centric relation, the case will usually be a failure.*

4. If the patient is wearing both upper and lower dentures, the lower denture is removed. Determine the rest position and the correct vertical relation using the appropriate procedure.[2]

[2] Described in Chapter 33.

5. The lower denture is reinserted in the mouth. Check the rest position and vertical relation, with the patient's old dentures in the mouth, against the correct rest position and vertical just recorded.[1]

6. The entire mouth is thoroughly examined for any undercuts, soreness, sharp, spinous ridges, and bulbous areas. Notation is made of their location. If undercuts are present and somewhat exaggerated, they must be removed.

7. A short medical history is taken, and record is made of any drug therapy the patient is currently undergoing. The name of his physician is noted.

Both husband and wife are present at the second appointment. At least an hour is allowed so that the case can be discussed in detail. The shortcomings, as well as the profound benefits, of dentures are thoroughly explained to both parties. Stress is placed upon the mental attitude the patient must cultivate in order to wear dentures successfully.

[1] Described in Chapter 34.

2

Preliminary Impressions

After the preliminaries—the sessions for consultation and evaluation, including the making of X-rays and study models, palpations of the hard and soft tissues, check of muscle spasms, and so on—have been attended to, we can proceed to the construction of upper and lower dentures. We begin with the preliminary impressions.

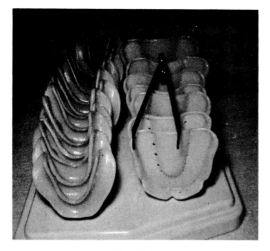

Fig. 2-1

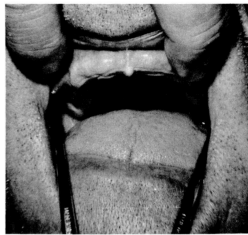

Fig. 2-2

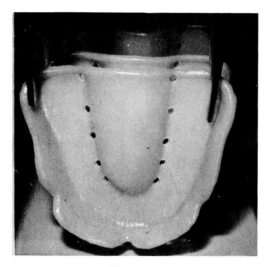

Fig. 2-3

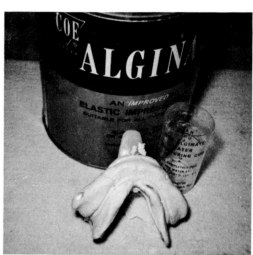

Fig. 2-4

Preliminary Upper Impression

1. At this point the Schreinmakers kit[1] (or an equivalent set-up) is made ready (Fig. 2-1). With the measuring calipers provided in the kit (Fig. 2-2), measure the distance between the buccal aspect of the maxilla in the region of the third molar on one side of the mouth to the same point on the opposite side of the mouth. The measurement is always taken on the buccal aspect from side to side at

the widest point of the maxilla. This affords the selection of a tray (Fig. 2-3) that will fit better from buccal-to-buccal surface than a tray selected arbitrarily.

2. Try the tray of choice in the mouth in order to verify the fit.

3. For impression material the author prefers Coe alginate (Fig. 2-4), although any heavy-bodied alginate can be used. Shake the alginate in the can thoroughly. Then measure out two full scoops of alginate into a rubber bowl.

[1]Imported by John Lust. Bonvini Dental Laboratory, 4695 Main St., Bridgeport, Conn. 06606.

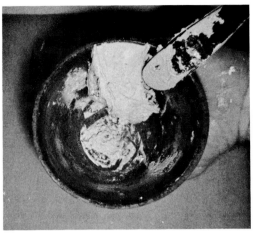

Fig. 2-5

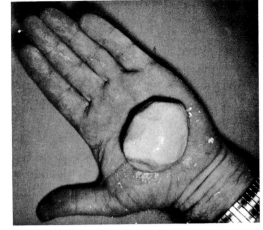

Fig. 2-6

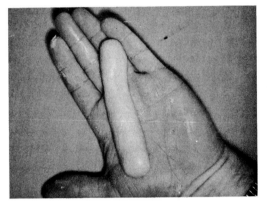

Fig. 2-7

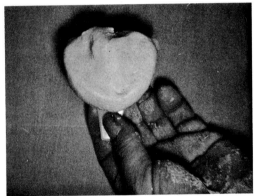

Fig. 2-8

4. Add 30 cc. tap water, and, with a heavy spatula, mix the water and alginate (which will be somewhat heavy) for one minute (Fig. 2-5).

5. Remove the mass from the rubber bowl with the spatula.

6. Dry hands and place this mass into palm and roll into a ball (Fig. 2-6) and then into a sausage shape (Fig. 2-7).

7. Now place this role of alginate into the acrylic tray and distribute it thoroughly (Fig. 2-8).

8. The patient's mouth should be opened wide to permit the introduction of the tray, and once the tray has been introduced, the mouth should be closed half way.

9. With vibrating motion, the tray is seated in place and held lightly with an index finger against the roof of the tray.

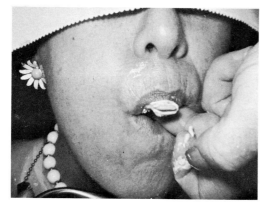

Fig. 2-9

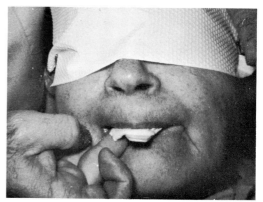

Fig. 2-10

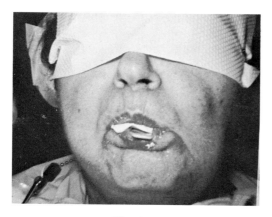

Fig. 2-11

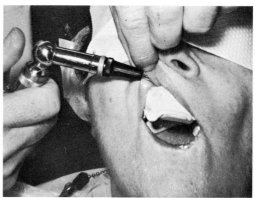

Fig. 2-12

10. As soon as the tray is seated, have the patient go through facial gymnastics—the motions of kissing (Fig. 2-9), grinning (Fig. 2-10), and moving the mandible from side to side (Fig. 2-11). This last step allows for the proper lateral movement of the coronoid process of the mandible, and will also provide the preliminary border height, which determines the thickness of the buccal border in the region that comes in contact in lateral movement of the coronoid process of the mandible. In many instances this step is overlooked, which may be a

cause of subsequent dislodgement of the upper denture.

11. After 3 minutes, remove the upper preliminary impression by having the patient blow with the lips closed; or you may use an air syringe (Fig. 2-12).

12. To avoid distortion of the alginate, pour up this impression immediately in any stone composition (Fig. 2-13). (Boxing is not necessary.)

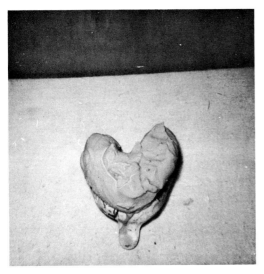

Fig. 2-13

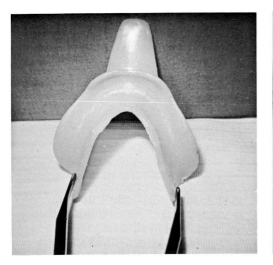

Fig. 2-15

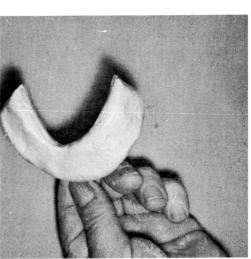

Fig. 2-16

Preliminary Lower Impression

1. With the calipers, measure the space between the lingual aspect of the retromolar pad on one side of the mouth to the same point on the other side of the mouth (Fig. 2-14).

2. Select an acrylic tray of proper width, as determined with the calipers (Fig. 2-15). Always measure the tray from lingual aspect to lingual aspect, as was done in the mouth.

3. Follow Steps 2 through 7 as given for upper preliminary impression.

4. Once the alginate has been mixed and placed firmly in the tray selected (Fig. 2-16), put the tray in the mouth and have the patient close half way.

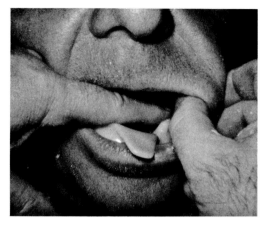

Fig. 2-17

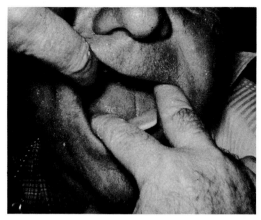

Fig. 2-18

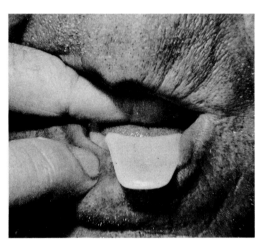

Fig. 2-19

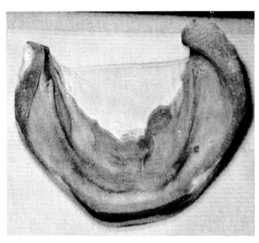

Fig. 2-20

5. Press one side to place; while holding the tray with the forefinger of the left hand (Fig. 2-17), manipulate the cheek in a rotary motion (for muscle trimming) with the thumb and forefinger of the right hand.

6. Now press the tray to place on the opposite side by holding it down with the thumb on the outside of the jaw and the forefinger on the tray. While doing so, manipulate cheek with the left hand (Fig. 2-18).

7. Upon completion of muscle trimming, use the forefinger holding the tray to strad-dle the finger rests on opposite sides of the tray (Fig. 2-19), and have the patient push the tongue slightly under that finger. This will give you a record of the correct physiologic length of the structures at the floor of the mouth.

8. After 3 minutes, remove the alginate impression from the mouth by use of an air syringe under its periphery and immediately pour up the impression using any good artificial stone (Fig. 2-20).

With preliminary impressions in hand, we proceed to the fabrication of acrylic trays.

3

Pouring Preliminary Impressions; the Construction of Acrylic Impression Trays

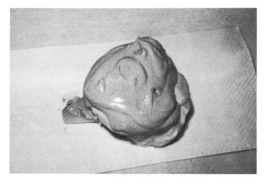

Fig. 3-1

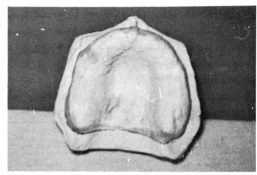

Fig. 3-2

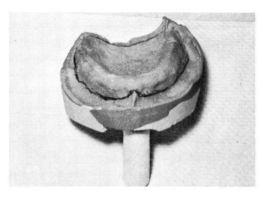

Fig. 3-3

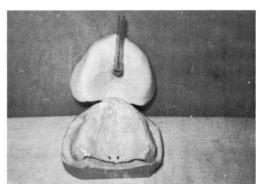

Fig. 3-4

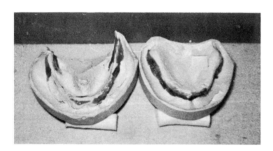

Fig. 3-5

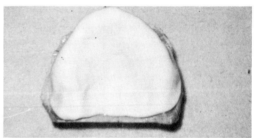

Fig. 3-6

When pouring preliminary impressions, invert them with the stone up (Fig. 3-1). This prevents the stone from falling away from the impression. (It is not necessary to box these impressions.) When the stone has set (Fig. 3-2), separate the stone cast from the impression. You are now ready to make the trays.

Upper Impression Tray Construction

1. Outline the preliminary cast with a soft pencil (Fig. 3-3) 2 mm. short of the muco-buccal fold, from hamular notch to hamular notch. For the fabrication of trays used in the posterior region, a line should be drawn from notch to notch about 2 to 3 mm. posterior to the fovea palatini (Fig. 3-4).

2. You may now eliminate undercuts with soft wax (Fig. 3-5).

3. Make the upper tray with any fast tray acrylic; no spacer is necessary (Fig. 3-6).

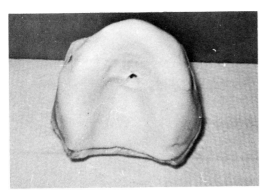

Fig. 3-7

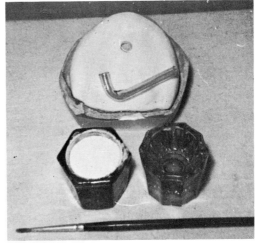

Fig. 3-8

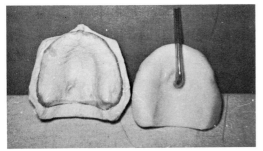

Fig. 3-9

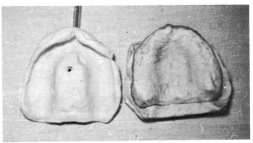

Fig. 3-10

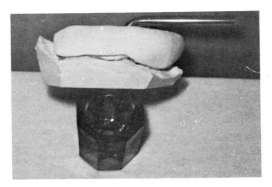

Fig. 3-11

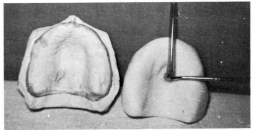

Fig. 3-12

4. When the tray acrylic is adapted over the model, and while the resin is still soft, with a round instrument, such as a small ball burnisher, make a hole in the area of the incisive palatine (Fig. 3-7) or in the center of the palate. Into this hole will be introduced the end of a manifold (Fig. 3-8) employed in the next step.[1]

5. Imbed a manifold (Figs. 3-9 and 3-10) made of tray tubing that has been softened in hot water and to a virtual 90 degree angle (Fig. 3-11).

6. Use powder and liquid resin to reinforce the manifold tube on the tray (Fig. 3-12).

[1] See Vacustatic Manual by American Precision Metals.

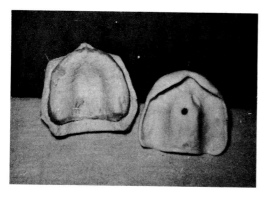

Fig. 3-13

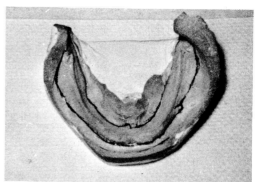

Fig. 3-14

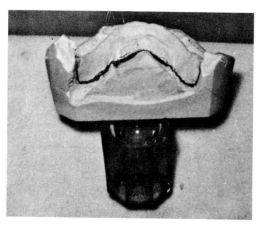

Fig. 3-15

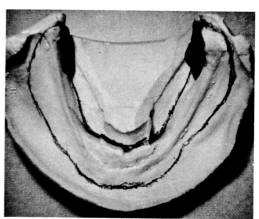

Fig. 3-16

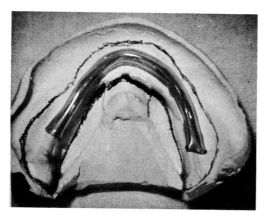

Fig. 3-17

Lower Impression Tray Construction

1. Outline the preliminary cast with a soft pencil (Fig. 3-14) 2 mm. short of the mucobuccal fold, from the buccal side of retromolar pad on one side to same point on the other side, and, similarly, from mucolingual fold to mucolingual fold (Fig. 3-15).

2. Eliminate undercuts with plastercine or soft wax (Fig. 3-16).

7. Trim the tray to the outline of the cast. This gives you the finished tray (Fig. 3-13).

3. In hot water, soften a length of manifold tubing and bend it to conform to the lower ridge, from second molar to second molar (Fig. 3-17).

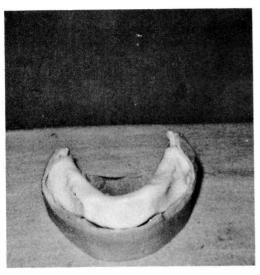

Fig. 3–18

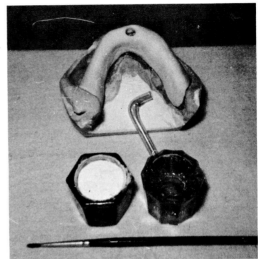

Fig. 3–19

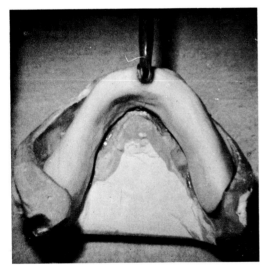

Fig. 3–20

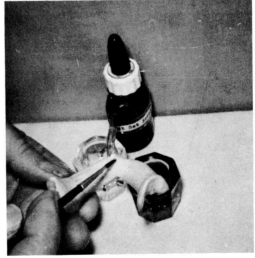

Fig. 3–21

4. Make a tray over the tubing and the cast with any fast tray acrylic (Fig. 3–18).

5. While the acrylic is still soft, make a hole through it for the manifold to reach the tubing on the cast (Fig. 3–19).

6. Insert the manifold, bent in hot water to a 90 degree angle, so that it reaches the tubing arched along the lower ridge (Fig. 3–20).

7. With acrylic powder and liquid, secure the manifold tubing to the tray (Fig. 3–21).

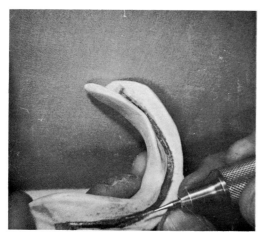

Fig. 3–22   Fig. 3–23

8. With a No. 700 bur, cut a channel in the tubing imbedded in the inner side of the tray from second bicuspid area to second bicuspid area (Fig. 3–22).

9. Trim the tray to the outline of the cast (Fig. 3–23).

4
Wash Impressions

It is always advisable to try-in the specially constructed upper and lower acrylic trays in the patient's mouth in order to ascertain a loose fit before proceeding with the actual wash impression procedure. The Vacu-static machine[1] is a significant aid in determining denture borders (Fig. 4-1).

In the following pages, wash impressions are made by two alternative methods, both satisfactory.

[1] American Precision Metals. 1801 Murchison Drive, Burlingame, California 94010.

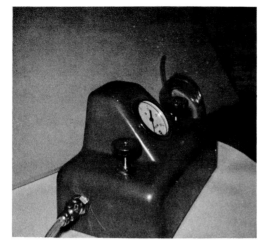

Fig. 4–1

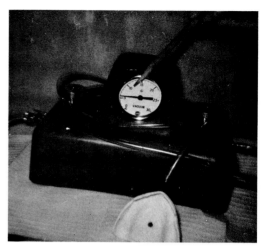

Fig. 4–2

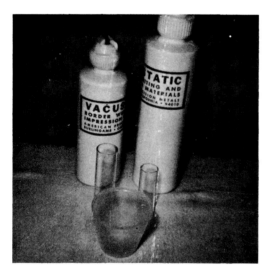

Fig. 4–3

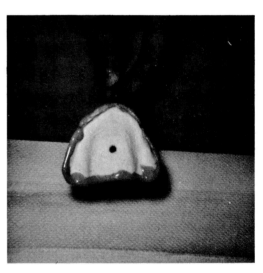

Fig. 4–4

USING A PLASTIC WAX AS A FINAL WASH

Upper Impressions

1. Make the appropriate connection of the Vacustatic machine to the saliva ejector of your dental unit and connect the 4-foot accessory tubing to the acrylic tray, setting the vacuum on the machine at 5 inches of pressure (Fig. 4–2).

2. Mix one portion of Vacustatic liquid and 2 portions of Vacustatic powder (Fig. 4–3) for 20 to 30 seconds in a plastic receptacle.

3. Immediately apply this mixture as a bead all the way around, and on, the periphery of the impression tray (Fig. 4–4).

4. Insert the tray in the patient's mouth and have him do mouth gymnastics, first sucking on the tube extending from the tray, next going through the motions of

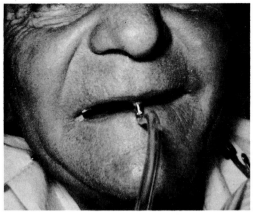

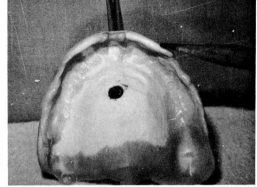

Fig. 4-5

Fig. 4-6

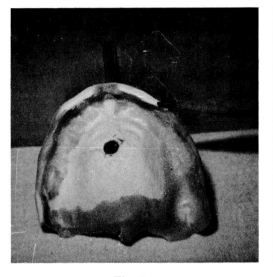

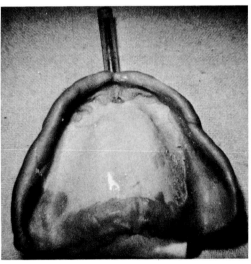

Fig. 4-7

Fig. 4-8

kissing and grinning, and, finally, moving the jaw from side to side (Fig. 4-5). During this procedure it is not necessary for the operator to support the tray. This is accomplished by the 5 inches of vacuum. The sucking, kissing and grinning motions afford rather accurate muscle trim, and waggling the lower jaw from side to side gives the proper trim of the coronoid process in the region of the buccal tuberosity.

5. After 3 minutes of mouth gymnastics, remove the tray from the mouth and examine it for overextensions (Fig. 4-6).

6. Trim off overextensions (Fig. 4-7).

7. Repaint the tray as before with a new mix of Vacustatic liquid and Vacustatic powder and insert it in the mouth.

8. Have the patient perform the same gymnastics as in Step 4.

9. After 3 minutes, re-examine the tray. If it is satisfactory, with no peripheral areas uncovered (Fig. 4-8), you are ready

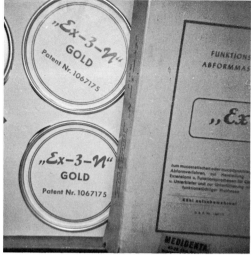

Fig. 4–9

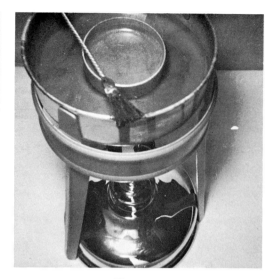

Fig. 4–10

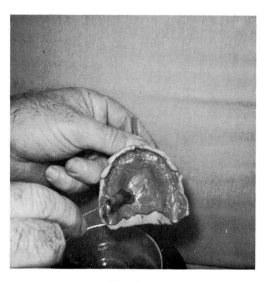

Fig. 4–11

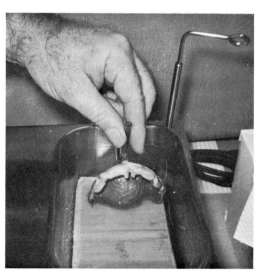

Fig. 4–12

to place a soft plastic wax, Ex-3-N[2] (Fig. 4–9), on the inside of the impression tray, which completes the wash impression procedure.

10. The Ex-3-N is first heated using a gas or alcohol lamp as per Ex-3-N kit instructions (Fig. 4–10) until it has melted to the consistency of heavy cream.

11. Using a brush, coat the previously rimmed Vacustatic tray with the melted wax, keeping away from the periphery (Fig. 4–11).

12. Place the tray in water heated to approximately 120°F. for 3 or 4 seconds (Fig. 4–12).

[2] Medidenta. 40–28 58th St., Woodside, N.Y. 11377.

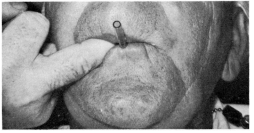

Fig. 4–13

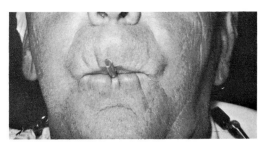

Fig. 4–14

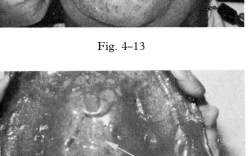

Fig. 4–15

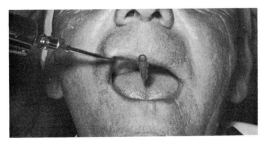

Fig. 4–16

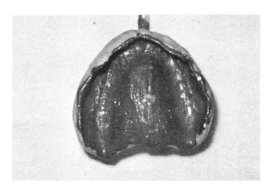

Fig. 4–17

15. The impression is released by having the patient balloon out his cheeks (Fig. 4–14).

16. Examine for underextension due to insufficient wax (Fig. 4–15).

17. Add more wax wherever necessary.

18. Place back in mouth for one minute.

19. Have patient perform slight gymnastic movements.

20. Pour ice cold water around the entire tray before removing it (Fig. 4–16).

21. Have the patient blow out the impression by ballooning his cheeks. The upper wash impression has now been completed (Fig. 4–17).

22. Pour the impression in stone immediately.

13. Place the tray in the patient's mouth, holding it in place with a finger of the right hand, exerting slight pressure upward (Fig. 4–13).

14. Maintain this pressure for one minute and have the patient perform slight gymnastic movements. (The Vacustatic machine may be used during this procedure.)

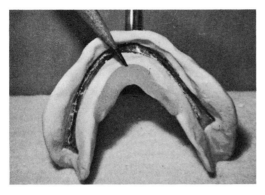

Fig. 4–18

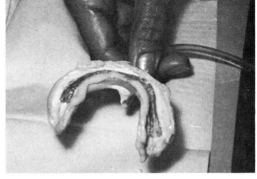

Fig. 4–19

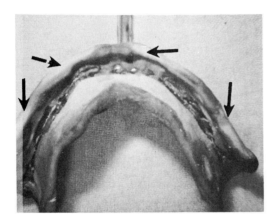

Fig. 4–20

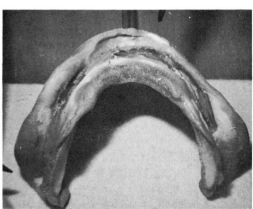

Fig. 4–21

Lower Impression

1. Try-in the lower acrylic tray in patient's mouth before proceeding with the wash impression procedure.

2. Apply Surgident peripheral wax lingually from the second bicuspid to second bicuspid (Fig 4–18), heat slightly with alcohol torch, insert in mouth and instruct patient to extend tongue slightly forward.

3. Attach the tray to the Vacustatic machine and set the vacuum at 5 inches of pressure.

4. Mix one portion of Vacustatic liquid and 2 portions of Vacustatic powder for 20 to 30 seconds.

5. Using a brush or spatula, apply this mixture as a bead all the way around the peripheral borders of the impression tray from the retromolar area on the buccal aspect to the retromolar area on the lingual aspect (Fig. 4–19).

6. Insert the tray in the patient's mouth and have him do mouth gymnastics—sucking on the extended tube, the motions of kissing and grinning. If the lower ridge is badly resorbed it may be necessary to hold the tray down with the index fingers of both hands.

7. After 3 minutes of mouth gymnastics, remove the tray from the mouth and examine it for overextensions (Fig. 4–20).

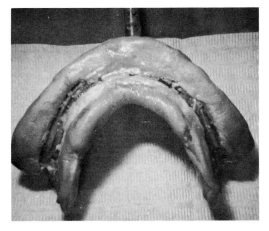

Fig. 4-22

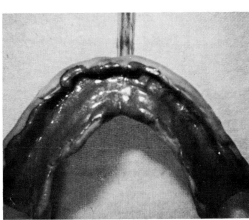

Fig. 4-23

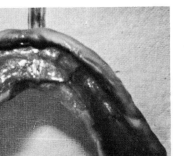

Fig. 4-24

Fig. 4-25

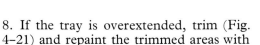

8. If the tray is overextended, trim (Fig. 4-21) and repaint the trimmed areas with a new mix of Vacustatic material.

9. Reinsert the tray in the mouth.

10. Direct the patient through the same gymnastics as in Step 6.

11. After 3 minutes re-examine the tray. If it is satisfactory and if the periphery is completely covered (Fig. 4-22) proceed to place Ex-3-N material (Fig. 4-23) on the inside of the impression tray.

12. Place the loaded tray in the patient's mouth and hold down on the lower ridge very lightly with the forefingers of each hand, stabilizing the hands by the thumbs under the chin.

13. At the end of one minute, and while holding lightly, have the patient perform the gymnastics of sucking, grinning, and slightly extending the tongue forward and pressing it against the area of the central incisors. This tongue action gives the correct raise to the structures in the floor of the mouth.

14. Remove the tray and examine it for insufficiency of material (Fig. 4-24).

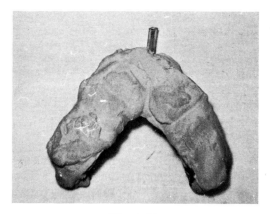

Fig. 4-26

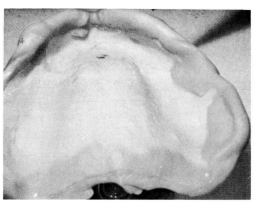

Fig. 4-27

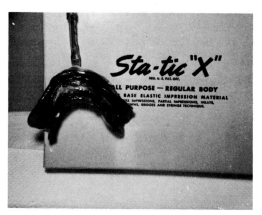

Fig. 4-28

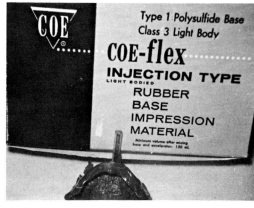

Fig. 4-29

15. Add Ex-3-N if necessary.

16. Dip the tray in water heated to approximately 120° F. for 3 or 4 seconds.

17. Reinsert in the mouth. While holding the tray with light pressure, have patient repeat the mouth gymnastics for one minute.

18. Before removing the impression from the mouth chill it thoroughly with ice water. This completes the procedure for the lower wash impression (Fig. 4-25).

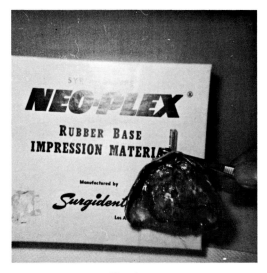

Fig. 4-30

19. Pour the impression in stone immediately (Fig. 4-26).

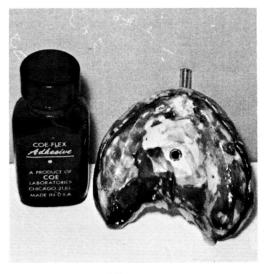

Fig. 4–31

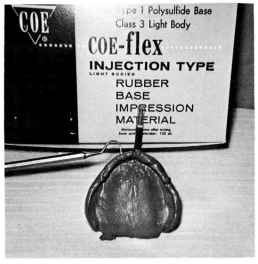

Fig. 4–32

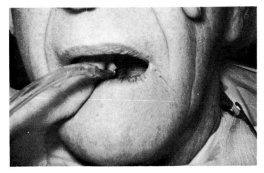

Fig. 4–33

Fig. 4–34

USING A RUBBER BASE AS A FINAL WASH

Upper Impressions

Repeat steps 1 to 8 on pages 18 and 19.

9. At the end of 3 minutes, re-examine the tray with the Vacustatic periphery. If it is proper (Fig. 4–27), you are ready to use a rubber base material such as Sta-tic-"X" (Fig. 4–28), Coe-Flex (Fig. 4–29) or Neo-Plex (Fig. 4–30).

10. Before using any of these, however, it is advisable to coat the entire inside of the tray, and the area over the Vacustatic ma-

terial, with Coe elastic cement (Fig. 4–31) or Sta-tic elastic cement. This assures better adhesion of the rubber base to the tray. It has been my experience that whichever rubber base material is used, provided it is mixed to a thin consistency, the resulting wash impression does not alter the height of my previously established peripheral borders (as determined by testing the thickness of the periphery with an explorer) (Fig. 4–32). I have found that although the material has flowed over the borders, it is paper-thin in those areas.

11. After thoroughly spatulating the rubber base on a paper mixing pad, spread it on the inside of the tray (Fig. 4–33).

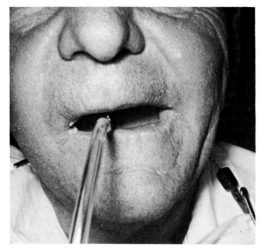

Fig. 4–35

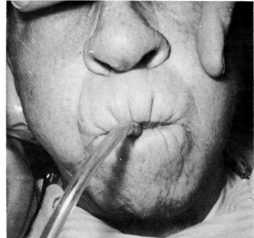

Fig. 4–36

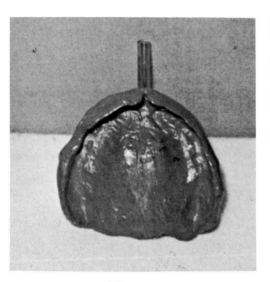

Fig. 4–37

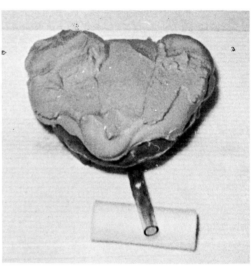

Fig. 4–38

12. Place the tray in patient's mouth and vibrate into place.

13. While holding the tray in place with the index finger of one hand, with very light upward pressure (Fig. 4–34), have the patient go through slight gymnastic movements.

14. It is advisable to use the Vacustatic machine during the taking of this wash impression (Fig. 4–35).

15. Remove the impression from mouth by having the patient balloon out his cheeks (Fig. 4–36).

16. Examine the impression to make sure there is a sufficient coverage of rubber base material. As a rule, the impression will be satisfactory (Fig. 4–37). This completes the upper wash impression.

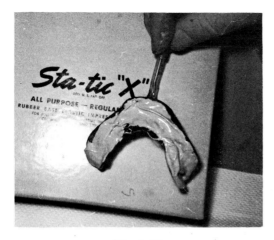

Fig. 4–39

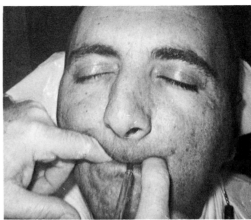

Fig. 4–40

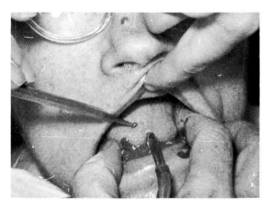

Fig. 4–41

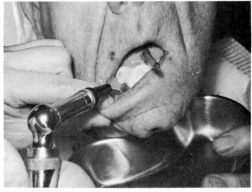

Fig. 4–42

17. Pour the impression upside-down in stone immediately (Fig. 4–38).

Lower Impressions

1. Repeat steps 1 through 10 as for upper wash impressions.

2. After thoroughly spatulating the rubber base on a paper mixing pad, spread on the inside of the tray (Fig. 4–39). For a lower ridge exhibiting significant movable tissue, I prefer to use Neo-Plex rubber base. It flows more easily and therefore offers less chance of distorting tissue.

3. Place this loaded tray in the patient's mouth and hold down on the lower ridge very lightly with the forefingers of each hand while applying thumb(s) under the patient's chin to stabilize your hands (Fig. 4–40).

4. Have the patient go through the gymnastics of sucking and grinning, and then have him slightly extend his tongue by pressing against the imaginary area of the lingual part of the lower central incisors. This tongue action gives the correct elevation to the structures in the floor of the mouth (Fig. 4–41).

5. Remove the impression from the mouth by using an air syringe under the periphery (Fig. 4–42).

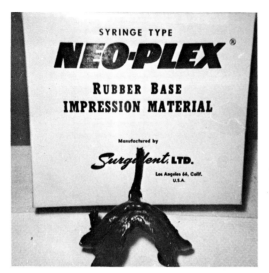

Fig. 4–43

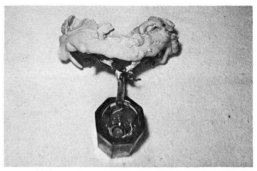

Fig. 4–44

6. Examine the finished impression (Fig. 4–43).

7. Pour impression upside-down in stone immediately (Fig. 4–44).

5
Building Bite Blocks from Wash Impressions

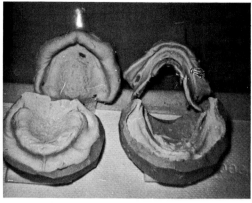

Fig. 5–1

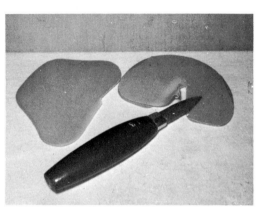

Fig. 5–2

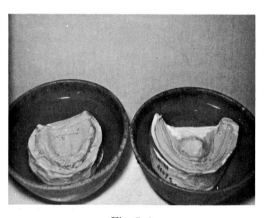

Fig. 5–3

Fig. 5–4

After the impressions have been separated (Fig. 5–1), we proceed to build bite blocks on the casts. If shellac trays are reinforced by coat-hanger wire and lined with plastic wafers[1] (Fig. 5–2), they are sturdy enough for the construction of wax rims and will withstand the recording of centric and eccentric occlusion. The trays are built according to the following procedure.

Upper Bite Blocks

1. First, it is necessary to moisten the stone model in water (Fig. 5–3).

2. Back a single-thickness base plate with a plastic wafer (Fig. 5–4).

[1] Stalite, Inc.

3. Heat the base plate backed with the wafer over the stone model until the mass drapes over it (Fig. 5–5).

4. Adapt the mass to the model with a moistened finger (Fig. 5–6).

5. Roll the mass around the periphery to the mucobuccal folds.

6. Insert the coat-hanger wire across the post-dam area (Fig. 5–7), keeping 4 to 5 mm. short of the posterior border in case shortening in this area is necessary.

7. Trim off the excess tray borders on a lathe, using sandpaper disks.

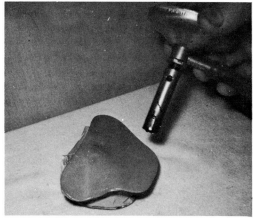

Fig. 5-5

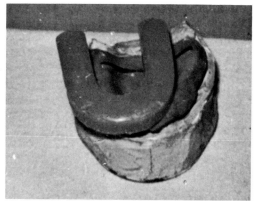

Fig. 5-6

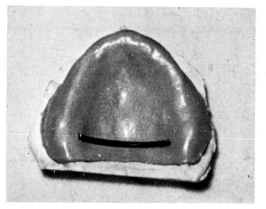

Fig. 5-7

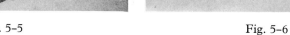

Fig. 5-8

8. Place hard wax bite forms[2] over the ridge from second molar to second molar (Fig. 5-8).

9. Using a hot spatula, seal this wax rim to the tray.

10. Complete the seal by using a hard sheet wax.

11. Cut away some of the plastic wafer from the post-dam area (Fig. 5-9). (This facilitates later checking in the post-dam

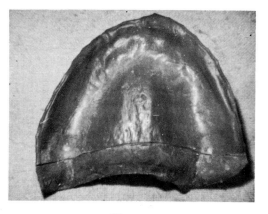

Fig. 5-9

[2] Modern Materials.

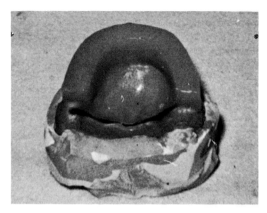

Fig. 5-10

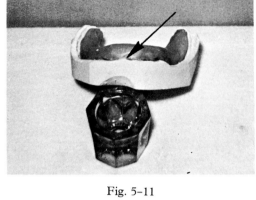

Fig. 5-11

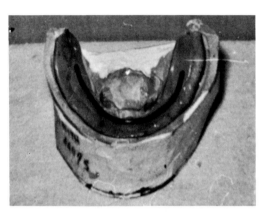

Fig. 5-12

area.) We now have a finished bit block (Fig. 5-10).

Lower Bite Blocks

The procedure for mandibular bite blocks is the same as that described for maxillary bite blocks, with one exception—a very low rim of hard wax is placed on the tray (Fig. 5-11) so that a soft wax can be superimposed at the time of recording vertical and centric relation. The mandibular bite block should be reinforced with coathanger wire on the lingual aspect from retromolar area to retromolar area (Fig. 5-12).

6

Preliminary Steps to Recording Vertical and Preliminary Centric Relation Through the Act of Swallowing

During the patient's first visit, when signs and symptoms were evaluated, we determined whether there was muscle spasm. If there was, we noted exactly where these areas of spasm existed. It is best to check these areas of possible spasm again, and to inject each with a 2 per cent local anesthetic having no vasoconstrictor action. Remember, however, that it is not the local anesthetic *per se* that breaks the spasm, but the puncture of the needle. The small amount of local anesthetic prevents needle pain as we make several punctures in a one-half-inch circle in the area of spasm.

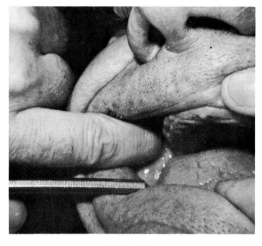

Fig. 6-1

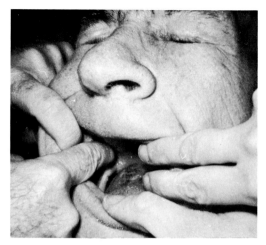

Fig. 6-2

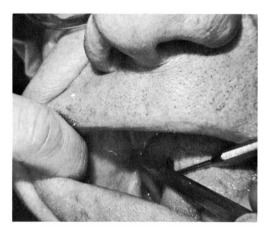

Fig. 6-3

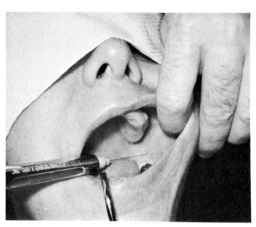

Fig. 6-4

THE TECHNIC OF BREAKING MUSCLE SPASM

1. After checking the attachments of the internal pterygoid muscle with the first finger of the left hand (Fig. 6-1), in the same region and in the same manner as one would palpate for a mandibular injection, apply light pressure medially just above the lingular bony prominence and observe whether the patient exhibits pain. [If a spasm is present it is usually unnecessary to ask the patient whether he feels pain; just watching his eyes as he winces (Fig. 6-2) tells us that he does.] In check-ing for spasms in the internal pterygoid region one must remember to stay away from any sharp lingula, so as to avoid a false response to the pressure applied (Fig. 6-3).

2. If we find that this area is in spasm, in-ject by syringe, using a 27 gauge dispos-able needle, a carpule of 2 per cent local anesthetic having no vasoconstrictor action (Fig. 6-4). Inject 2 drops of the anesthetic to a depth of about 2 mm.

3. If the opposite side is affected, repeat the same procedure.

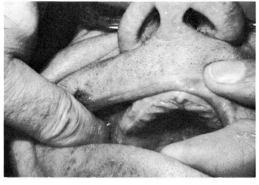

Fig. 6-5

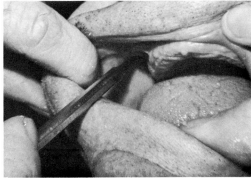

Fig. 6-6

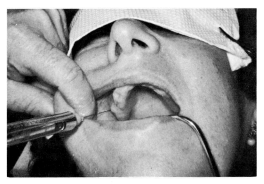

Fig. 6-7

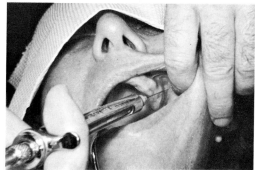

Fig. 6-8

4. Now recheck to determine whether the fibers of the external pterygoid muscle are in spasm. [They are found in the area of the maxilla high up (Fig. 6-5) on the fold above and in back of the third molar.] Apply pressure medially with the first finger (Fig. 6-6).

5. If spasm is present on both sides, inject (Fig. 6-7) both sides of the mouth in the same manner as was done for the internal pterygoids (Fig. 6-8) of the mandible (see Step 1).

6. Now go back over all the muscle areas previously checked. Using only the point of the needle, form a one-half-inch circle of punctures in each. This helps to break the spasms completely.

IMPORTANCE OF BREAKING MUSCLE SPASM

Why are these spasms so important, and why must they be eliminated before we attempt to record vertical and centric relation? All of us, I am sure, have had the unfortunate experience of recording centric relation by one method or another, and then, after having had the laboratory set up the teeth, of finding at the "try-in" that we had missed the "bite." We then placed wax over the lower set-up, had the patient retrude (or we gently retruded) the mandible, and took another registration for a reset. When this reset was ready for try-in we found that we still had the wrong centric relation. The next time we might have removed the lower set-up, placed wax over the areas, and positioned the mandible for another reset—only to find a third time that it did not check out.

Now we had become somewhat disturbed. At this juncture, some of us might have become more sophisticated and have placed a central bearing in the set-up, taking a gothic arch centric. Now we were *sure* that we had the correct centric relation, only to find at the try-in that it was still not correct. How disappointing, and how frustrating. In desperation we moved the teeth around in the mouth for interdigitation and sent the case to the laboratory for processing.

This case was doomed to failure—because vertical and centric relation were not right and never would be, owing to spasms that were present, were unrecognized, and were never released.

Only recently a patient complained to me of constant discomfort in both mandible and maxilla. He had been wearing a full upper denture and a partial lower denture for nearly four years. The mandibular partial denture replaced three anterior teeth and two bicuspids on one side and the second bicuspid and first molar on the other. This left him with two good molars, cuspid and lateral, on one side, and cuspid, first bicuspid and second molar on the other side. The remaining teeth, from a peridontal point of view, were in good condition.

In my opinion, a fixed prosthesis should have been resorted to in the mandible in the first place; however, the type of restoration was not the cause of the pain. From the symptoms he gave, it was evident that he suffered from temporomandibular joint dysfunction. And confirmation of this came upon palpation of the internal and external pterygoid muscle fiber attachments. He reacted strenuously, almost bolting from the pain in those areas.

7

Determination of Correct Anterior Length and the Placement of the Post-Dam in the Upper Bite Block

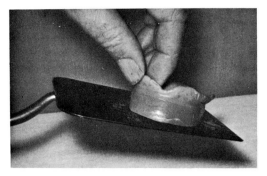

Fig. 7-1

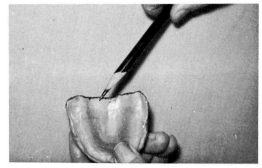

Fig. 7-2

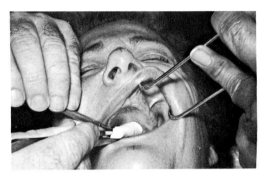

Fig. 7-3

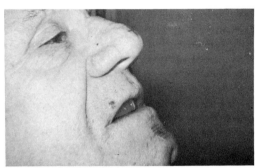

Fig. 7-4

When all muscle spasms have been relieved, you are ready to record vertical and centric occlusion. First establish the correct occlusal height by use of a hot plate to reduce wax length (Fig. 7-1). Then establish the correct length of the bite block and the placement of the post-dam area in the following manner.

Occlusal Height

If the patient who comes to us edentulous has photographs showing the former profile of his teeth, they are a great aid in determining the length of the upper anterior bite block. However, if there are no pre-extraction photographs or records showing the extent to which the patient displayed his natural teeth, we are forced to determine the length of the upper bite block by other means.

One guide to determine how much of the teeth to show is the age of the patient—the older the patient, the less teeth we will show (and the shorter the bite block); the younger the patient, the more teeth we will show (and the longer the bite block).

Post-Dam Area

The post-dam area should always be established by the dentist and not by the dental technician. I do not believe in using the fovea palatinae as a means of determining the length of the denture because the fovea palatinae are sometimes anterior, and sometimes posterior, to the point at which the denture should end. Therefore, if you ask your technician always to build the posterior portion of the bite block a little longer than necessary, you can establish the correct length yourself. This is done in the following manner.

1. With an indelible pencil, mark well the entire distal end of the bite block (Fig. 7-2) on the palatal side from tuberosity to tuberosity, which will come in contact with the palate when placed in the mouth.

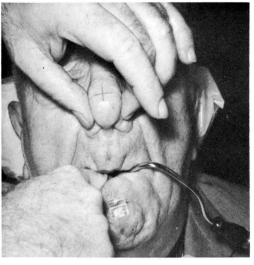

Fig. 7-5

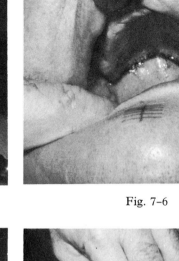

Fig. 7-6

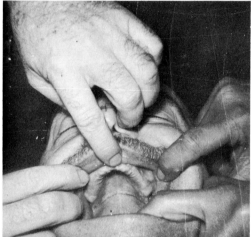

Fig. 7-7

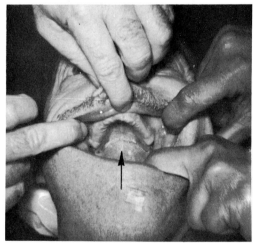

Fig. 7-8

2. Using a cotton roll, dry the patient's palate (Fig. 7-3).

3. Insert the marked bite block into the patient's mouth (Fig. 7-4).

4. While holding the patient's nose with two fingers of one hand, and while holding down the tongue with one or two fingers of your other hand, in order to avoid the tongue's obliterating the marking (Fig.

7-5), have him blow his nose. This causes the palate to descend and contact the pencil marking on the bite block, leaving traces of this mark across its distal portion (Fig. 7-6).

5. Remove the bite block while still holding down the patient's tongue (Fig. 7-7).

6. Place your two fingers on his nose and ask him to blow his nose again (Fig. 7-8).

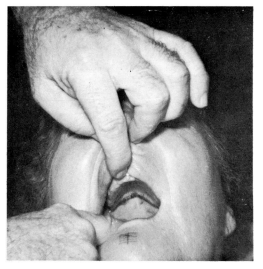

Fig. 7–9

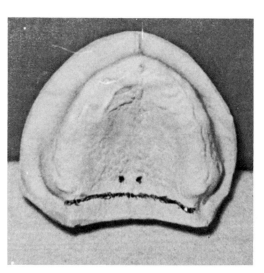

Fig. 7–10

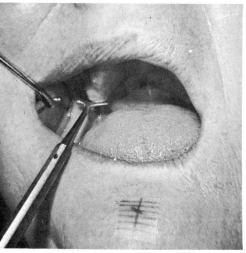

Fig. 7–11

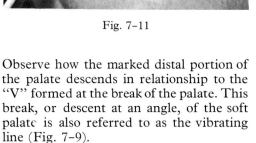

Fig. 7–12

Observe how the marked distal portion of the palate descends in relationship to the "V" formed at the break of the palate. This break, or descent at an angle, of the soft palate is also referred to as the vibrating line (Fig. 7–9).

7. If your original marking was too long, too far toward the throat and therefore away from the vibrating line, cut the bite block back until it is 1.5 to 2.0 mm. past the vibrating line.

8. If the bite block is anterior to the vibrating line, extend it until it is about 1.5 to 2.0 mm. past the vibrating line.

9. Transfer the corrections in length made on the bite block to the model (Fig. 7–10) and, with a No. 1 bur, cut in on the model the distal extent of the bite block from tuberosity to tuberosity.

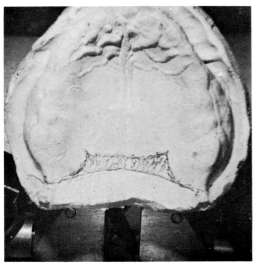

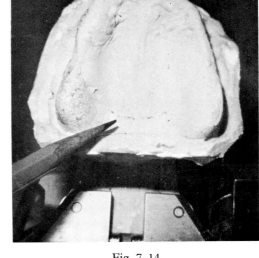

Fig. 7–13

Fig. 7–14

10. Now, to locate the area over the hamular notch, the following procedure is employed: Start skidding a T burnisher from the molar ridge area back toward the throat (Fig. 7–11). As you keep going back you literally fall off the cliff; as you continue to skid back, you will feel another drop-off. End the denture bite block at the second drop-off.

11. Make a notation of this point on your stone model (Fig. 7–12).

12. Palpate with a ball burnisher the amount of movable tissue present in the mouth between the two hamular notches in order to be able to approximate (Fig. 7–13) the amount the model may be scraped in the post-dam area to create a better seal between the denture and the palate. At the extreme distal end (Fig. 7–14) it may be scraped deeper and gradually lessened as we come forward anteriorly. As we scrape the model we try to follow the anatomy of the hard palate at that point.

8
Determination of the Occlusal Plane

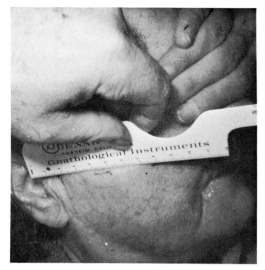

Fig. 8–1

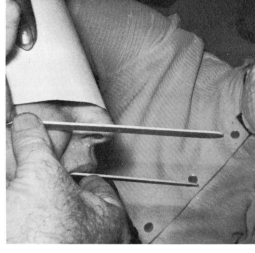

Fig. 8–2

The occlusal plane, as defined in a glossary of prosthodontic terms is, "an imaginary surface which is related anatomically to the cranium and which theoretically touches the incisal edges of the incisors and tips of the occluding surfaces of the posterior teeth. It is not a plane in the true sense of the word but represents the mean of the curvature of the surface."

It is the author's experience that the determination of the occlusal plane (which will be determined more accurately in Chapter 12) is very important. If the occlusal plane as it pertains to the lower denture is raised or lowered too much, the patient may experience difficulty in removing the food from the occlusal table, and therefore help to dislodge the lower denture, or bite the lateral borders of the tongue.

After establishing the anterior length on our bite block, a workable arbitrary occlusal plane is now established. This is done in the following manner.

Using the fixed points of the tragus of the ear (Fig. 8–1) and the ala of the nose as landmarks, we try by means of tongue depressors or a Fox gauge to establish a line from the posterior to the anterior part of the bite block as parallel as possible to the tragus-ala line. Many times it will be necessary to shave off the wax on the posterior occlusal surface of the bite block until a state of parallelism (Fig. 8–2) between the tragus-ala line and the bite block is achieved.

After completing this procedure and making sure that spasms have been eliminated, we can record vertical and preliminary centric relation.

9

The Recording of Vertical and Preliminary Centric Relation Through the Act of Swallowing

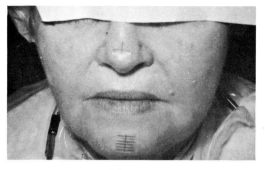

Fig. 9–1

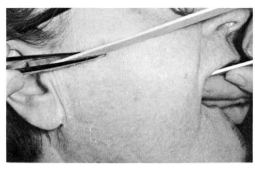

Fig. 9–2

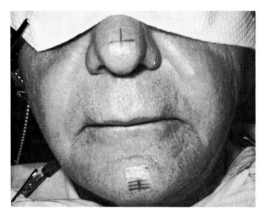

Fig. 9–3

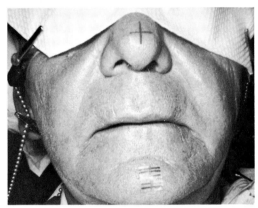

Fig. 9–4

1. Place one piece of tape marked with "+" on the tip of the patient's nose and a second, marked with a vertical line intersected by 4 or 5 horizontal lines (spaced about 2 mm. apart), on his chin (Fig. 9–1).

2. Place in his mouth the upper bite block, which will have been adjusted to the correct lip line, correct post-dam length and to the tragus-ala occlusal plane (Fig. 9–2).

3. Ask the patient to sit erect and to lick his lips while repeating the word "Emma." He should relax and should ignore your movements while you are taking measurements.

4. When you know that the patient is relaxed (Fig. 9–3), and while he is saying "Emma" and his lips are slightly apart (Fig. 9–4), measure with calipers the distance between the "+" on the nose and the uppermost horizontal line on the chin (Fig. 9–5). This distance indicates the "rest position" of the mandible. Actually, the rest position when teeth are present is revealed by the distance or space between the teeth when the jaws are apart.

5. Once you have determined the rest position (which should be verified by repeating the measurement several times), determine the free-way space. This is done in the following way.
   a. While holding one end of the calipers on the nose mark "+" and the other end slightly away from, not touching, the chin markings (⅛ in. is adequate clearance), ask the patient to swallow.
   b. Observe at the "peak" of the swallow

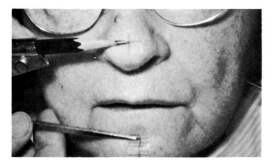

Fig. 9–5

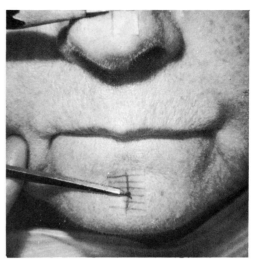

Fig. 9–6

which horizontal mark on the chin is aligned with the end of the caliper (Fig. 9–6). (Because at this time there is no lower bite block in the mouth, he will swallow upward, toward the nose mark, without interference.)

c. By counting the horizontal marks crossed during the act of swallowing, you can determine easily how many millimeters of free-way space the patient needs. An old-fashioned but unfortunately still popular belief is that a 3 mm. free-way space is universally adequate. I have observed patients exhibiting adequate free-way spaces of 5, 7, 9, 11 and 13 mm. Furthermore, it has been my experience that if an individually inadequate free-way space is not recognized and provided, the case will be a failure. If we do not allow for an adequate space, nature will attempt to provide one at the expense of the underlying structures.

We must measure free-way space accurately and not rely only on appearance and approximations. The fact that the upper and lower bite blocks look well and fill out the mouth does not imply necessarily that the free-way space is adequate. It is well known that an open or a closed vertical, especially the former, causes temporomandibular joint symptoms and the problems that go with them.

I recommend that the measurement described here for determining the correct free-way space be re-

peated several times to insure accuracy. After some practice you will be gratified to find that you are able to record this free-way space over and over again and obtain the same results each time.

To recapitulate, what does the measurement of the range of motion during swallowing really mean? Simply that the lowermost horizontal line reached by the caliper during the swallow reveals the patient's jaw closure when, with the lower bite block in the mouth, he contacts the upper bite block. In other words, it is in this position and at this point that the patient's upper and lower teeth contact during the last stage of deglutition. When his jaws open and he assumes the rest position again, the distance between the jaws constitutes the free-way space. Thus, the free-way space is the amount of space that should be present between the jaws when they are apart in physiologic rest.

6. Once you have recorded by means of the calipers the rest position on the chin

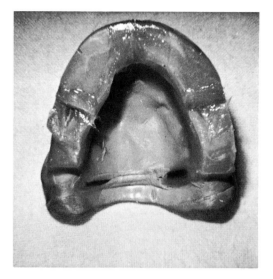

Fig. 9–7

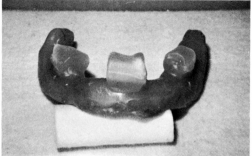

Fig. 9–8

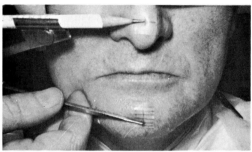

Fig. 9–10

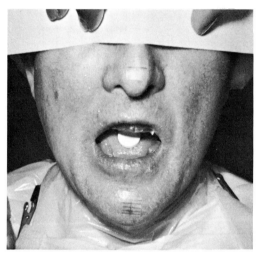

Fig. 9–9

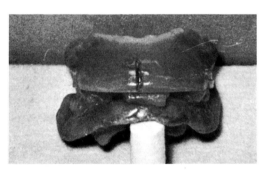

Fig. 9–11

(Fig. 9–7), key the upper bite block in the right and left molar and anterior regions, applying ample petrolatum to all three regions.

7. Place three mounds (Fig. 9–8) of soft wax[1] on the lower bite block (lute well), opposite the keys of the upper bite block.

8. Heat the wax mounds slightly with an alcohol torch.

9. Lightly powder the upper and lower bite blocks with a good adhesive.

10. Insert in the patient's mouth.

[1] Wafer Wax by Modern Materials.

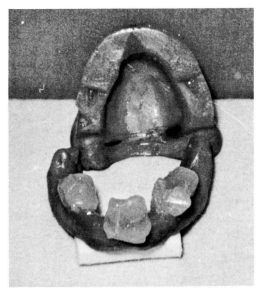

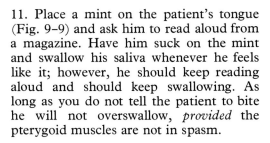

Fig. 9–12

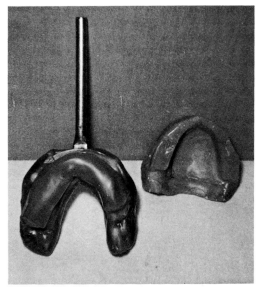

Fig. 9–13

11. Place a mint on the patient's tongue (Fig. 9–9) and ask him to read aloud from a magazine. Have him suck on the mint and swallow his saliva whenever he feels like it; however, he should keep reading aloud and should keep swallowing. As long as you do not tell the patient to bite he will not overswallow, *provided* the pterygoid muscles are not in spasm.

12. After about 5 to 10 minutes of reading and swallowing, check the nose and chin marks and note his progress (Fig. 9–10). In almost every case you will notice that the patient has swallowed in the correct previously established vertical relation (see Fig. 9–6). Also, he has given us a fairly accurate hinge centric relationship.

13. Thoroughly chill with ice water both the upper and lower bite blocks to which the three mounds of wax had been attached in Step 7.

14. Remove the bite blocks from the mouth (Fig. 9–11) and separate the upper bite block from the lower one (whose wax attachments now appear indented) (Fig. 9–12).

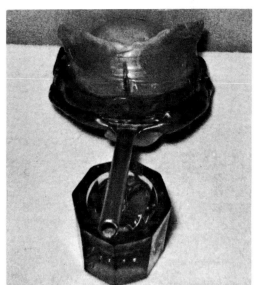

Fig. 9–14

15. Envelop the bite fork of an articulator[1] (Fig. 9–13) in a medium-hard set-up wax and insert the keyed upper bite block into the prepared fork (Fig. 9–14).

[1] Whip Mix Articulator, Whip Mix Corp., Louisville, Ky.

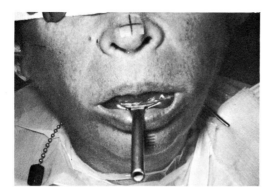

Fig. 9–15

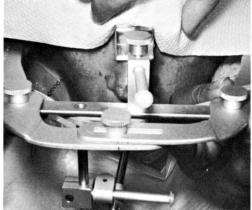

Fig. 9–16

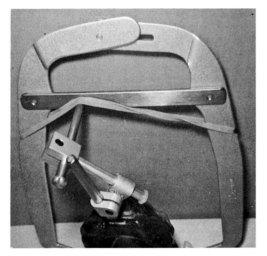

Fig. 9–17

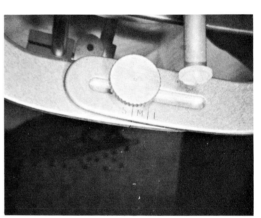

Fig. 9–18

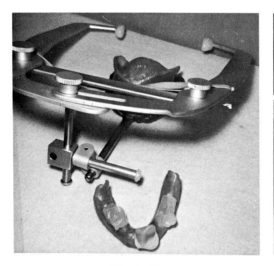

Fig. 9–19

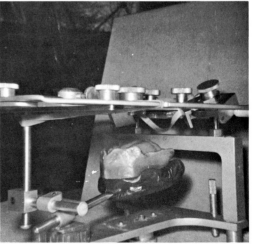

Fig. 9–20

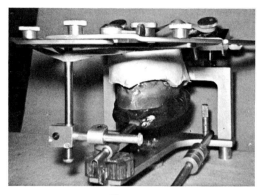

Fig. 9-21

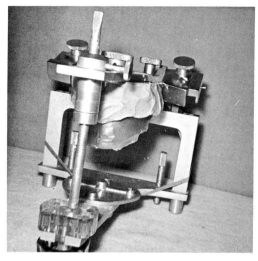

Fig. 9-22

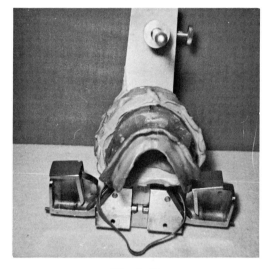

Fig. 9-23

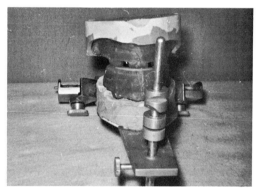

Fig. 9-24

16. Take this to the mouth (Fig. 9-15), and using a face bow[1] (Fig. 9-16), make a record (Fig. 9-17). While taking this face bow record observe the marking of the intercondular distance directly in front of the face bow (designated "S" for short, "M" for medium, and "L" for large) (Fig. 9-18). (Use of the articulator is covered in detail in Chapters 15 and 18.)

17. After thoroughly securing the face bow instrument to the bite fork, remove it from the mouth (Fig. 9-19).

18. Mount this face bow record on the articulator (Fig. 9-20).

19. Articulate the upper cast to the articulator by means of a stone composition (Fig. 9-21).

20. When the stone has set, remove the face bow apparatus (Fig. 9-22).

21. Fit the wax-indented lower bite block to the keyed upper bite block (Fig. 9-23).

22. Insert the lower cast into the lower bite block (Fig. 9-24).

[1] Whip Mix Corp.

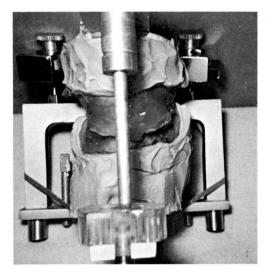

Fig. 9–25

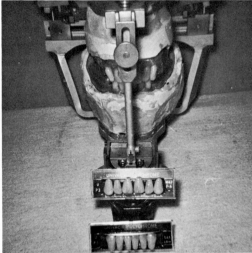

Fig. 9–26

23. Finish the articulation (Fig. 9–25).

24. The six upper and lower anterior teeth (Fig. 9–26) are set up at this time using Pound's[1] principles.

25. The selection of teeth and their placement on the dental arches is discussed in Chapters 10, 11 and 12.

[1] E. Pound: Esthetics and phonetics. J. Prost. Dent., Oct. 1966.

10

Shaping the Upper Bite Block as an Aid in Setting the Upper Six Anterior Teeth

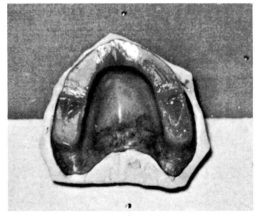

Fig. 10-1

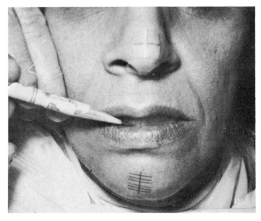

Fig. 10-2

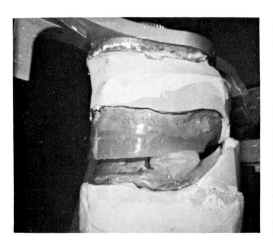

Fig. 10-3

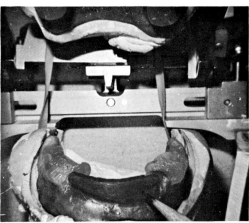

Fig. 10-4

SHAPING THE ANTERIOR WAX FOR POSITIONING THE UPPER SIX ANTERIOR TEETH

During the establishment of the tentative occlusal plane we determined approximately the anterior lip length of the maxillary bite block. Now the anterior section of this wax bite block can be shaped from cuspid to cuspid region (Fig. 10-1), and this should be done in such a way as to conform to the wet-dry line of the lower lip when the patient says the letter "F" (Fig. 10-2). In other words, keep cutting or adding wax to this segment until the wax lightly contacts the wet-dry line on the lower lip from cuspid to cuspid. If sufficient time is spent it is possible to contour the upper bite block so that the teeth can be positioned correctly from this contour. Nonetheless, when checking esthetics and phonetics, it may be necessary to make slight alterations in the positioning of the upper teeth so placed.

The Positioning of the Lower Six Anterior Teeth

After the upper anterior wax bite block has been adjusted we now turn our attention to the anterior section of the lower bite block.

1. First, remove the anterior soft wax stop (wafer wax; Fig. 10-3) that was used in

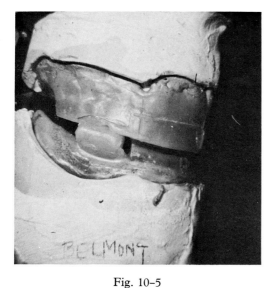

Fig. 10-5

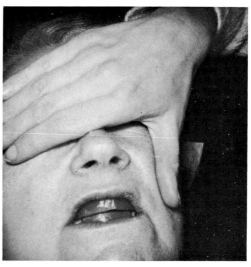

Fig. 10-6

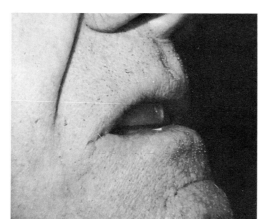

Fig. 10-7

Fig. 10-8

taking tentative vertical and centric relation.

2. Replace the wafer wax with a narrow red or white softer bite rim wax from cuspid to cuspid (Fig. 10-4), and have this wax contact the maxillary bite block on the case previous articulated that has the established vertical dimension (Fig. 10-5).

3. Now remove both bite blocks from the articulator and insert the wax rims into patient's mouth (Fig. 10-6).

4. Ask the patient to count from 60 to 70 several times. Observe as the patient pronounces the sound "S" how far the mandible moves forward (Fig. 10-7), if it moves at all. The more the mandible moves forward, the more overjet will be needed. In other words, the mandibular anteriors will be placed farther lingually in relation to the lingual surfaces of the maxillary anteriors (Fig. 10-8). Adjust the lower wax to this position.

For those who prefer not to employ this softer red wax for the correct positioning of the lower six anteriors, the same objective may be reached by shaping and bending the anterior wax of the lower bite block just prior to the swallow-in procedure when recording tentative vertical and centric occlusion.

The final test for phonetics and esthetics will usually determine the amount of overbite. However, for the initial six upper and lower trial set-up, a good rule is to introduce about the same degree of vertical overlap as was necessary in the horizontal overbite. The amount of overbite and overjet is usually referred to as "incisal guidance."

11
Selection and Setting of Anterior Teeth

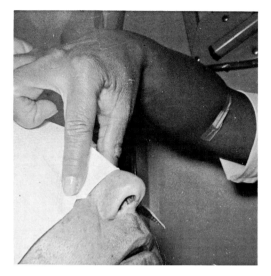

Fig. 11-1

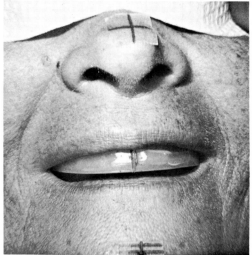

Fig. 11-2

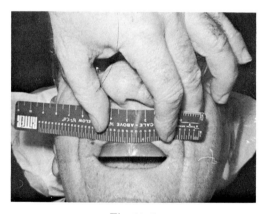

Fig. 11-3

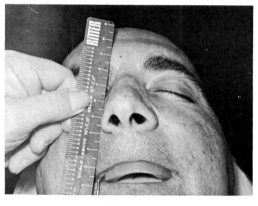

Fig. 11-4

There are many methods by which dentists have been selecting and setting teeth. I shall illustrate two methods that I believe aid in the setting of the upper and lower anteriors, and one method (in Chapter 12) of positioning the posteriors. (That method at the same time may help to correct, if biologically necessary, the original tentative occlusal plane taken by the tragus-ala landmarks.)

UNIVERSAL DENTAL CO. SELECTOR

The first method (advanced by the Universal Dental Co.[1]) incorporates a selector

[1]Mr. Joseph P. Kitchenman, Consultant, Universal Dental Co., Philadelphia, Pa.

to determine the mold for the proper length and width of the upper anterior teeth.

1. The previously correctly contoured and length-established upper wax bite block is reinserted in the mouth (Fig. 11-1).

2. The patient is asked to smile, and the height of the lip line is observed (Fig. 11-2). With the straight edge of a ruler, mark this "smile line" parallel to the incisal part of the bite block (Fig. 11-3).

3. Using the ruler, mark the distal of the

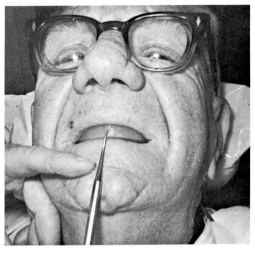

Fig. 11-5

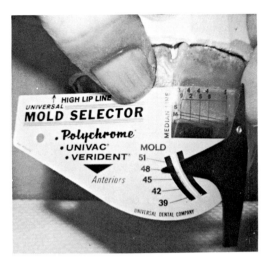

Fig. 11-6

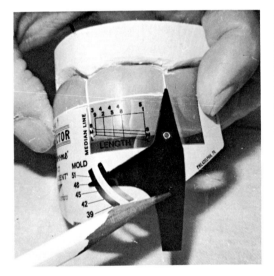

Fig. 11-7

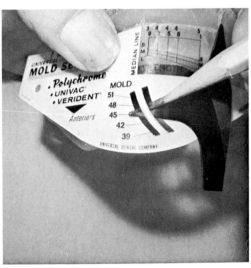

Fig. 11-8

cuspid areas on the bite block by placing the ruler in line with the lacrimal duct and the ala of the nose on both sides of the face (Fig. 11-4).

4. Mark the median line (Fig. 11-5).

5. By placing the mold selector and lining up the median line of the selector with the median line and high smile line of the bite block (Fig. 11-6), and by moving the scanner (Fig. 11-7) to the distal line of the cuspid, note that the other end of the scanner indicates the number of the mold required. Thus, the mold selector automatically gives you the width of the mold (Fig. 11-8). This mold selector, in addition to indicating the mold number for a specific case, also indicates the required length of that mold.

6. To determine the length of the mold (the mold number, or width, having been

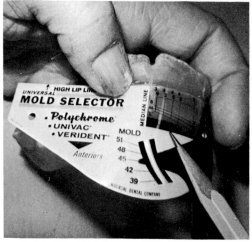

Fig. 11-9

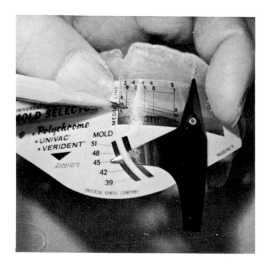

Fig. 11-10

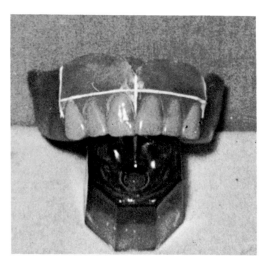

Fig. 11-11

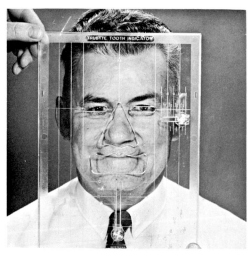

Fig. 11-12

selected as described above), read through the transparent area of the selector marked "length" (Fig. 11-9) at the point where the length line of the mold number (previously selected) intersects with the occlusal plane on the bite block. This will indicate the length of the mold required— L (long), M (medium), or S (short). In the instance shown, medium (M) length is indicated (Fig. 11-10).

7. After selecting the six upper anteriors we refer to the mold guide of the manu-

facturer for the selection of the corresponding lower anterior teeth. After the landmarks are established and the six upper and lower anterior teeth have been selected, it is a simple matter to place them in the pre-established areas (Fig. 11-11).

TRUBYTE SYSTEM

The second method used in anterior tooth selection (advanced by Dentists' Supply Co.[1]) is known as the Trubyte system.

[1] Courtesy of Mr. Herbert A. Bates, Dentists' Supply Co., York, Pa.

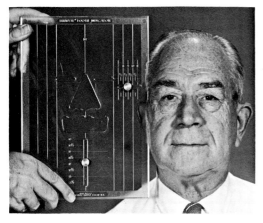

Fig. 11-13

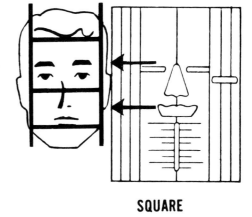

SQUARE

Fig. 11-14

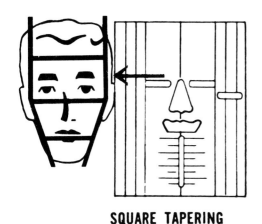

SQUARE TAPERING

Fig. 11-15

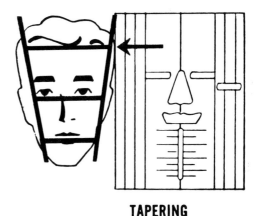

TAPERING

Fig. 11-16

The Trubyte tooth indicator (Fig. 11-12) can be used in one of two different ways to determine outline form.

1. In order to select the form of tooth that will harmonize with the outline form of the face, place the edge of the tooth indicator in a vertical position against the side of the patient's face and head, touching the side of his face just forward of the ear (Fig. 11-13).

Square Form

While in this position (Fig. 11-14), if the side of the tooth indicator touches from:
  a. A point ⅔ up the forehead (normally at the hairline)

  b. to the level of the condyle forward of ear and
  c. to the angle of the mandible, and if these lines are parallel on both sides, we have a square outline form.

Square Tapering Form

In this position (Fig. 11-15) if the edge of the indicator touches reference points
  a. ⅔ up the forehead to
  b. the level of the condyle, with the indicator held in a vertical position, and from reference point B [level of condyle to reference point
  c. (the angle of the mandible)] with indicator tilted inward and downward, we have the square tapering outline form.

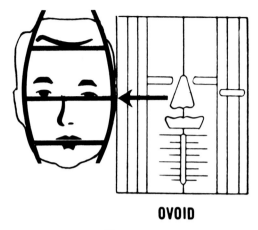

OVOID

Fig. 11-17

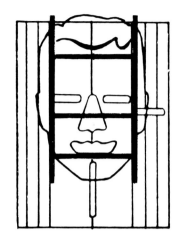

SQUARE

Fig. 11-18

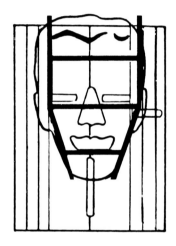

SQUARE TAPERING

Fig. 11-19

Tapering Form

If with side of the indicator placed just forward of the ear we find that it touches points A (⅔ up the forehead), B (the level of the condyle) and C (the angle of the mandible), with widest portion being at point A, we have a tapering form (Fig. 11-16).

Ovoid Form

1. If the indicator is held in front of the ear in a vertical position and is tilted upward and inward to point A (⅔ up the forehead), and then retilted from this same point (in front of ear) downward and inward to point C (the angle of the mandible), and we find that the widest portion is at the level of the condyles, we have the ovoid outline form (Fig. 11-17).

2. We can now use the tooth indicator by another method, which involves its positioning on the patient's face in such a manner that the horizontal slots of the indicator are level with the pupils of the patient's eyes, the instrument's vertical center line coinciding with the median line of the face.

Square Form

If when sighting through the inscribed vertical lines the sides of the patient's face approximately follow the vertical lines from points A (⅔ up the forehead), B (the level of the condyle) and C (the angle of the mandible), we have the square outline form (Fig. 11-18).

Square Tapering Form

If when sighting through the inscribed vertical lines the sides of the patient's face

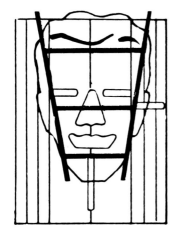

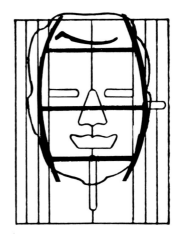

TAPERING

Fig. 11-20

OVOID

Fig. 11-21

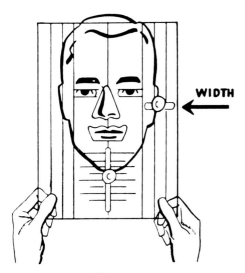

Fig. 11-22

from point A (⅔ up the forehead) to point B (level of the condyles) to point C (the angle of the mandible) taper inward, we have the tapering outline form. In this form the widest portion of the face would be at point A (⅔ up the forehead) (Fig. 11-20).

Ovoid Form

If when sighting through the inscribed vertical lines, we find that the widest portion of the face is through point B (level of the condyles) curving inward and upward to point A (⅔ up the forehead) and inward and downward to point C (the angle of the mandible), we have the ovoid outline form (Fig. 11-21).

Determining the Size of the Upper Anterior Teeth

1. Place the tooth indicator on the patient's face in such a manner that the horizontal slots of the indicator are level with the pupils of the patient's eyes, its vertical center line coinciding with the median line of the face.

Now move the upper indicator bar inward (Fig. 11-22) until tissue contact is made and lock in place. Next, bring the lower indicator bar upwards under the

from points A (⅔ up the forehead) and to B (the level of the condyles) approximately parallel the vertical lines of the indicator, and the sides of the face from point B (the level of the condyle) to point C (the angle of the mandible) taper inward, we have the square tapering outline form (Fig. 11-19).

Tapering Form

If when sighting through the inscribed vertical lines the sides of the patient's face

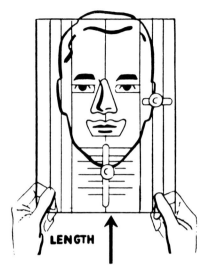

LENGTH

Fig. 11–23

chin until bony contact at the base of the chin is made (Fig. 11–23).

The width of the maxillary central is noted by observing the calibrations along the side of the upper indicator bar. It is the inner edge of this bar that determines the width of the central. Next observe the upper edge of the lower bar to determine the length of the maxillary central by observing the calibrations along the side of the lower indicator bar. This measurement is based on a 16 to 1 ratio between face size and tooth size.

Having now determined the outline form as well as the size (width and length) of the maxillary central, we turn to the mold chart and, being guided by the determined outline form, we check first for the desired width and then the length. Owing to the vertical space available in the mouth it might sometimes be necessary to modify the length of the tooth. However, the width usually remains constant.

Using this procedure in the selection of the maxillary central automatically gives us the width of the six anteriors. Matching the mold for the lower anteriors is suggested in the mold chart for the average normal case. However, it might be necessary to modify the selection in unusual cases.

While the Trubyte tooth indicator is not infallible, it is a useful modality. Its use also shows the patient that we are attempting a somewhat scientific approach to tooth selection.

Color Selection of Teeth

In color selection we find that people tending toward a darker complexion, and people with darker hair and darker eyes, usually have teeth that exhibit a certain over-all greyness, especially in the maxillary centrals. People with lighter complexions, the blue-eyed blond, tend to exhibit an over-all yellow band of color, particularly in the maxillary centrals. (A complete tooth color analysis guide is available from the Dentists' Supply Co.)

12

Esthetics and Phonetics; Determining the Position of the Lower Posterior Teeth

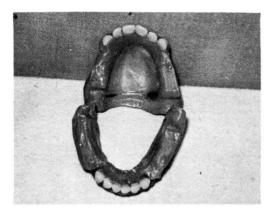

Fig. 12-1

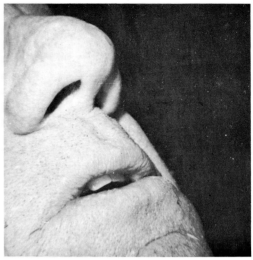

Fig. 12-2

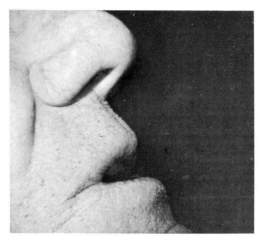

Fig. 12-3

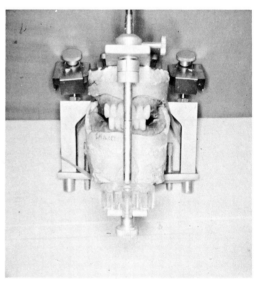

Fig. 12-4

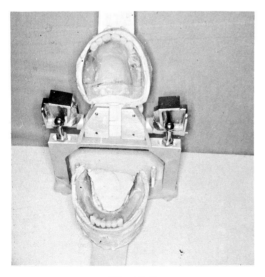

Fig. 12-5

CHECKING TRY-INS FOR ESTHETICS AND PHONETICS

With the six upper and six lower set-up on the bite blocks, we now check for esthetics and phonetics (Fig. 12-1).

1. To check for esthetics, insert these bite blocks into the patient's mouth and notice

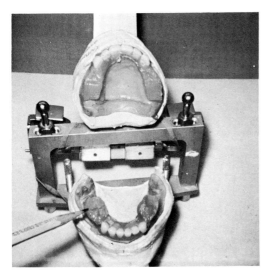

Fig. 12-6

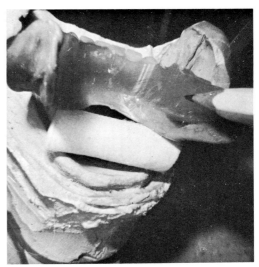

Fig. 12-7

whether the maxillary teeth fall on the inner wet-dry line of the lip when the patient pronounces the letter "F" (Fig. 12-2).

2. If any deviation is necessary, make corrections.

3. To check phonetics, have the patient count from 60 to 70 and when he utters the "S" sound (Fig. 12-3) notice whether there is sufficient overjet and no hissing, and that the teeth are not touching—that they are at least 1 mm. apart.

4. Have the patient approve the esthetics of the anterior teeth. At this juncture it is best to determine whether the spouse also approves.

POSITIONING THE LOWER POSTERIORS ON THE BITE RIM

If everyone is satisfied with the esthetics and phonetics at this time, we now prepare the mandibular bite block for the next step in the setting of the posteriors. The questions we ask are: What determines the setting? At what occlusal height, and in what position, are we to set the posteriors? There are many approaches to this problem. We have all heard the advice to set the posterior teeth on the ridge. Does this mean that we are to set the teeth where the ridge was or where it has settled—downward and inward—and thus perhaps interfere with the functions of the tongue? Or are we to set the teeth *off* the ridge—where the ridge *was*? And, if so, *where* off the ridge?

To answer these questions, we employ the following procedures.

1. After the six upper and lower anterior teeth have been set up (Fig. 12-4), remove the soft wafer wax in the molar regions from the mandibular rim (Fig. 12-5) and replace it with hard wax. This wax should be indented into the keys of the maxillary bite block (Fig. 12-6). This procedure maintains the vertical dimension during the next step, which consists of bringing the bite blocks together in contact and having the patient swallow, in order to record a lower tongue form.

2. Scoop out wax from the lingual surface of the mandibular bite block (Fig. 12-7) to allow for introduction of blue flange wax.[1]

[1] Surgident Co., Los Angeles, Cal.

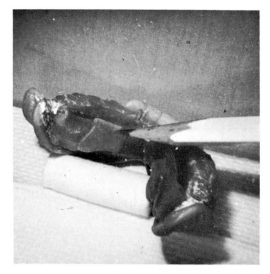

Fig. 12-8

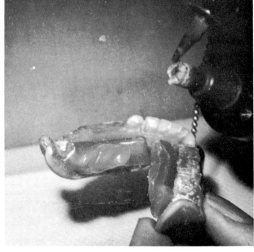

Fig. 12-9

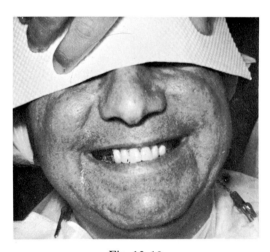

Fig. 12-10

3. Place flange wax on the entire lingual surface from the distolingual retromolar area on one side to the distolingual retromolar area on the opposite side (Fig. 12-8).

4. Place petroleum jelly on the maxillary teeth and surrounding areas.

5. Slightly heat the flange wax on the mandibular bite block with an alcohol torch (Fig. 12-9).

6. Replace both bite blocks (which have the six upper and lower anterior teeth setups) in the patient's mouth (Fig. 12-10).

7. Have him close in centric (into the posterior red wax indents) and start swallowing.

8. Have him keep his jaws together while swallowing, and press his tongue forward against the lingual surfaces of the mandibular anteriors.

9. After 3 minutes, remove the lower bite block and examine it for over- or underextension of the flange wax.

10. If there is a downward overextension (Fig. 12-11A), cut off the excess.

11. If there is not enough wax add more.

12. After 2 or 3 insertions and block examinations (and after you have determined that the tongue will not displace any more

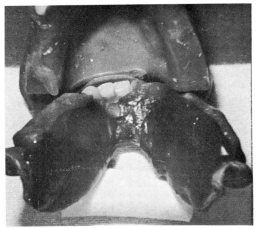

Fig. 12–11A

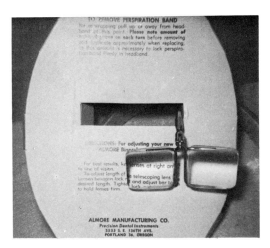

Fig. 12–11B

wax), chill the lower bite block thoroughly with ice water. Remove it and examine with binocular loops (Fig. 12–11B).[1]

13. If sufficient wax was introduced, a fine shiney demarcation line toward the upper border of the mandibular bite rim will be visible. Intensify this mark with a fine scribe line to preserve it (Fig. 12–12), and rub plaster or stone into it (Fig. 12–13).

14. This fine curling over of the flange wax was dictated by the lateral borders of the tongue, and it indicates the exact occlusal height and width at which the lingual cusps of the mandibular molars should be placed.

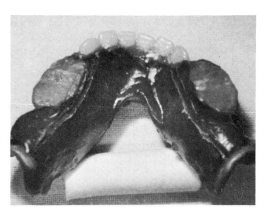

Fig. 12–12

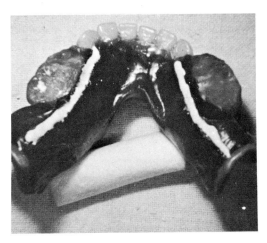

Fig. 12–13

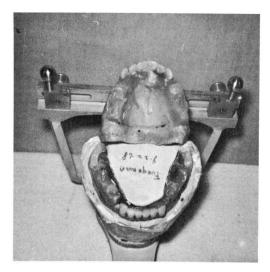

Fig. 12-14

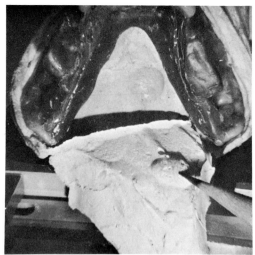

Fig. 12-15

15. Replace the lower bite block on the cast. After blocking out some of the lingual undercuts, pour the stone tongue index to the height of the scribed line (Fig. 12-14).

16. When the stone tongue index has hardened, removed the tongue form and flange wax (Fig. 12-15).

13

Mechanical Aids in the Recording of Centric and Eccentric Positions

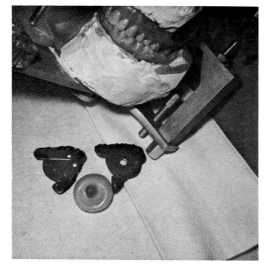

Fig. 13–1

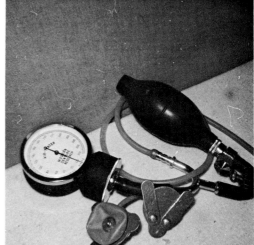

Fig. 13–2

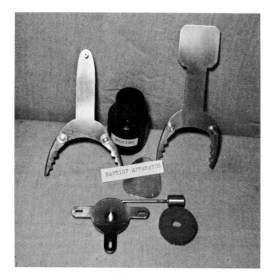

Fig. 13–3

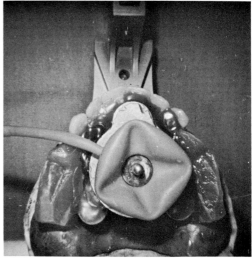

Fig. 13–4

For the dentist who wishes even greater refinement in his denture work, I suggest the use of any one of the following special intra-oral air-centric devices[1] (Fig. 13–1), or one of which includes a bulb-inflated air cushion and a shut-off valve for mainte-nance pressure (Fig. 13–2). One of the best is a simple, home-made, extra-oral-intra-oral appliance[2] (Fig. 13–3), or some similar ready-made apparatus, which utilizes a stylus and platform, and employs a rubber washer over the central bearing. This ap-

[1] Air-Centric Bite Technic, Modern Denture Research Co., Box 812, Santa Monica, California.

[2] Victor Baptist, 85 Leeuwarden Road, Darien, Connecticut, 06820.

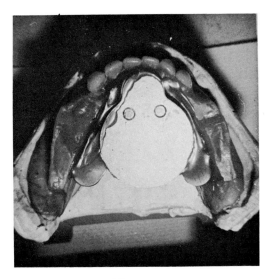

Fig. 13-5

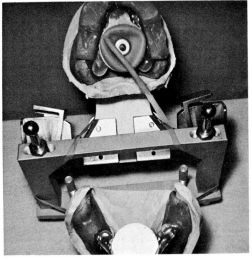

Fig. 13-6

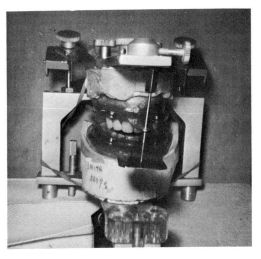

Fig. 13-7

paratus gives correct gothic arch centric and eccentric recordings that can be used in the registration of stone check bites. As the late Claude Stansbury demonstrated many years ago, a gothic arch tracing taken without an air bubble, or other device permitting the correct centering of the lower platform on the lower base in order to distribute the pressures to the center of tissue resistance, could result in centric and eccentric positions that are incorrect.

After preliminary centric of the six anterior maxillary and mandibular set-ups have been determined, proceed to the following:

1. Place the air-centric inflatable cushion into the vault of the maxillary bite set-up and secure with sticky wax (Fig. 13-4).

2. Place the platform on the mandibular try-in just beneath the occlusal and incisal areas of the teeth (Fig. 13-5), and secure with compound or sticky wax.

3. Open the pin on the upper apparatus (Fig. 13-6) so that the occlusion is opened about 3 mm. (Fig. 13-7). This will allow the patient freedom of movement during the recording of both centric and eccentric positions.

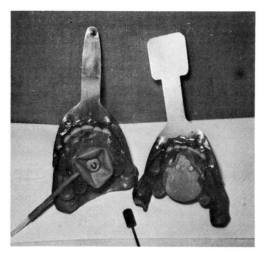

Fig. 13-8

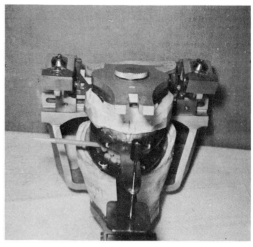

Fig. 13-9

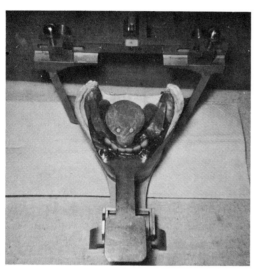

Fig. 13-10

4. Now place the upper extra oral jaw-like apparatus, which will hold the stylus, on the outside of the maxillary try-in set-up (Fig. 13-8) and secure with sticky wax.

5. Parallel to the upper apparatus, line up the lower extra oral apparatus, which will carry the lower recording platform on the six mandibular anteriors, and secure with sticky wax (Figs. 13-9 and 13-10).

14

Recording Centric Occlusion, Bennett Movements and Condylar Inclinations Under Air-Centric Gothic Arch Tracings

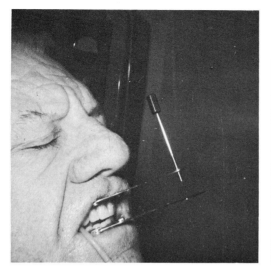

Fig. 14-1

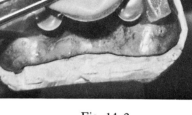

Fig. 14-2

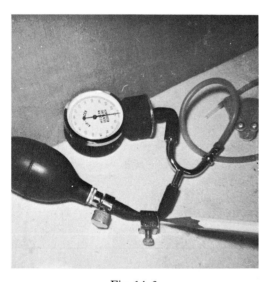

Fig. 14-3

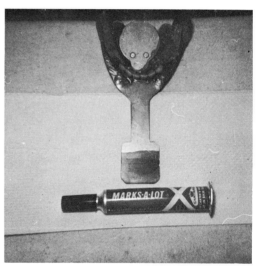

Fig. 14-4

1. Place the apparatuses (Chapter 13) into the patient's mouth and check for freedom of movement (Fig. 14-1). The central bearing screw (Fig. 14-2) should be opened about 3 mm. to permit the clearance of anterior teeth during movements.

2. Inflate the gauge to 140 to 220 mm. of pressure (Fig. 14-3) and have the patient practice centric and eccentric movements

prior to the actual recording of the gothic arch tracing.

3. Using a black or blue indelible pencil, coat the platform holding the mandibular try-in (Fig. 14-4).

4. Insert the pin into the stylus holder but hold pin up away from platform and have

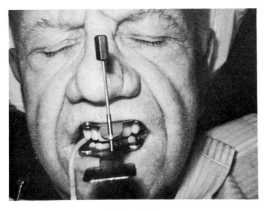

Fig. 14-5

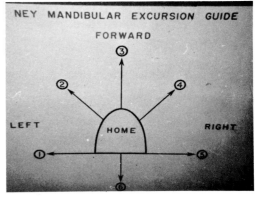

Fig. 14-6

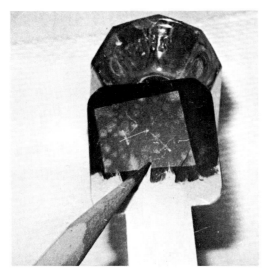

Fig. 14-7

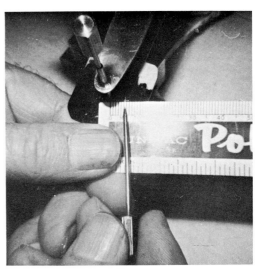

Fig. 14-8

the patient protrude and retrude several times, dropping pin down each time, making sure that he makes the same dot marking on the mandibular try-in each time (Fig. 14-5).

5. At this point, it is quite helpful to have him hold the Ney Mandibular Excursion Guides,[1] also known as the Flocken mandibular guide (Fig. 14-6). Repeat the mandibular movements. The numbers on the Guide help him to perform the centric and eccentric movements.

6. After the centric dot marking, have him scribe right and left laterals, and this will form the gothic arch tracing (Fig. 14-7).

7. With a ruler, measure off 6 mm. on these lateral lines (Fig. 13-8).

8. Place petrolatum on the six upper and lower teeth of these dentures.

[1] The Ney Co., Bloomfield, Connecticut.

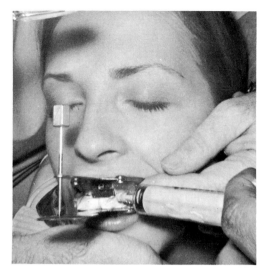

Fig. 14-9

Fig. 14-10

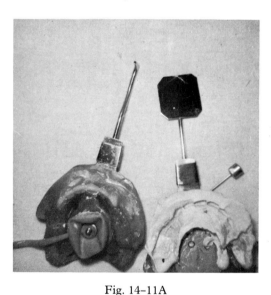

Fig. 14-11A

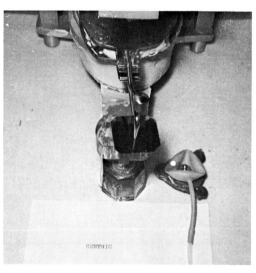

Fig. 14-11B

9. Have the patient hold in centric, and with a disposable plastic syringe[1] (Fig. 14-9) inject fast-setting Healey Gray Rock stone composition. Hold his chin so that his jaws remain in centric position. If this is done properly the pin does not move from the apex of the gothic arch tracing (Fig. 14-10).

[1] Monojet disposable syringe, Brunswick Labs., Deland, Florida.

10. When the stone has set, release the air pressure and remove from the mouth the upper and lower try-in dentures, with the interposed stone, either both dentures together or separated (Fig. 14-11A).

11. Reassemble the upper and lower try-in dentures to the centric stone index by first removing the central bearing apparatus from the palate. Place these assembled

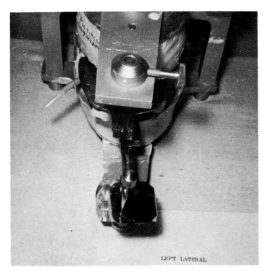

Fig. 14–12

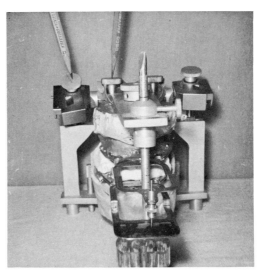

Fig. 14–13

dentures on the maxillary cast of the articulator and finish the articulation (Fig. 14–11B).

12. When the stone has set, remove the try-in apparatuses from the articulator and, replacing the central bearing apparatus, re-insert in the mouth in order to record left lateral position.

13. In recording the left lateral position, have him move his jaw to the previously marked 6 mm. point on the line, and while holding at this mark shoot in the stone with a syringe.

14. When the stone has set, release the air pressure, remove the entire stone locked-in apparatus from the mouth and place it in a Whip Mix articulator (Fig. 14–12). (Always set the opposite side of the instrument.)

15. Set Bennett and condylar inclinations of movement on the right side of the articulator (Fig. 14–13) and make a record of the readings, not only to achieve balance, but for regrinding and adjusting the occlusion later.

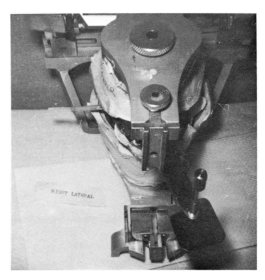

Fig. 14–14

16. Remove the apparatus from the articulator and place it back in the patient's mouth and record right lateral position using same procedure as for the left lateral. Secure this position with fast-set stone as was done in Steps 9 and 13.

17. When the stone has set, release the air pressure, remove the entire stone locked-in apparatus from the mouth and insert into the articulator (Fig. 14–14).

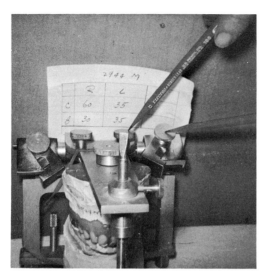

Fig. 14–15

18. Set the left side of the articulator for Bennett and condylar positions and record the readings (Fig. 14–15).

19. Protrusive recording is not necessary with this instrument.

In rechecking centric relation-occlusion with this procedure it has been my experience that the centric relation originally noted by the swallowing procedure is usually the same anteroposteriorly, but might be slightly different laterally. The difference is explained by the fact that the air appliance equalizes pressure on the ridges, and therefore fosters more accurate technic.

15

Setting Bennett Movements and Condylar Inclinations on the Whip Mix Articulator

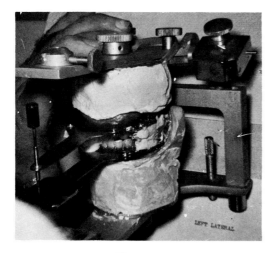

Fig. 15-1

Fig. 15-2

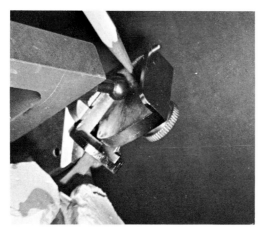

Fig. 15-3

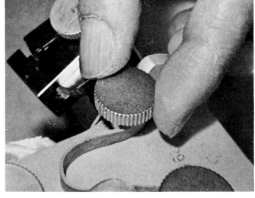

Fig. 15-4

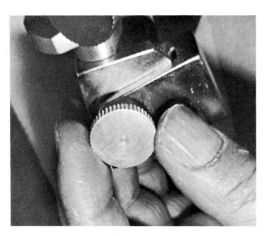

Fig. 15-5

After placing the left stone check bite in place in the articulator proceed to set the opposite, or right, side of the instrument.

1. When the instrument is first positioned (the upper and lower sections in contact) (Fig. 15-1) ascertain that the ball of the left condyle on the lower part of the instrument is in its socket (Fig. 15-2) and that the ball of the right condyle is away from its socket (Fig. 15-3).

2. On the right side, loosen up the condyle (Fig. 15-4) and Bennett screws (Fig. 15-5).

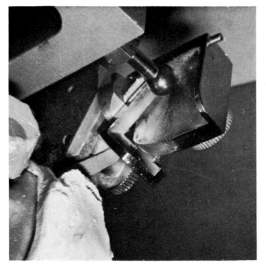

Fig. 15-6

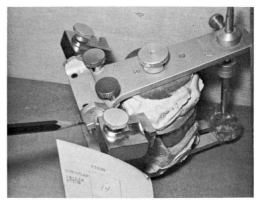

Fig. 15-7

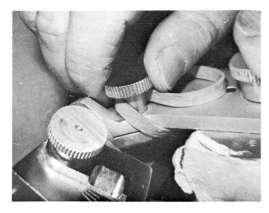

Fig. 15-8

Fig. 15-9

3. Set the condyle inclination by first tipping the box back (Fig. 15-6) and then bringing it down until it contacts the ball on the lower section of the articulator (Fig. 15-7). Now tighten the condyle screw (Fig. 15-8). While making these adjustments, be certain that the left condyle stays in place and does not move out of position.

4. Take the condylar reading (Fig. 15-9).

5. Adjust the Bennett movement by bringing the lever in the box socket over toward the inside of the articulator first (Fig. 15-10) and then gradually back away toward

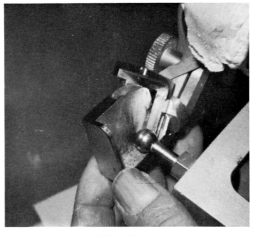

Fig. 15-10

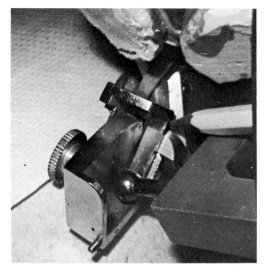

Fig. 15-11

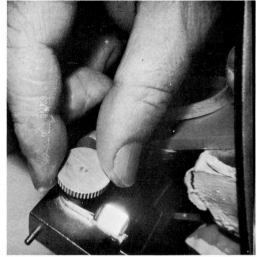

Fig. 15-12

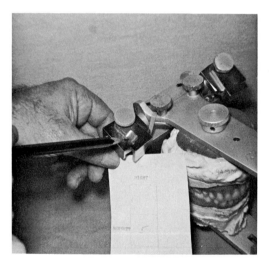

Fig. 15-13

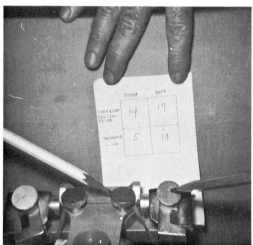

Fig. 15-14

the outside (or away from the articulator) until the mesial part of the ball is contacted (Fig. 15-11). Lock the screw (Fig. 15-12) and record the degree of Bennett movement (Fig. 15-13).

6. For setting the Bennett movement and condylar inclination for the right stone check bite, repeat this procedure on the opposite side of the articulator and record condylar inclination and Bennett movement (Fig. 15-14).

16
Positioning and Setting of Posterior Teeth

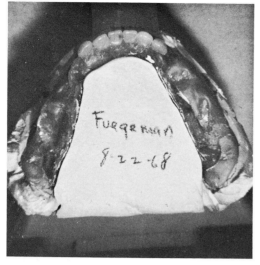

Fig. 16-1

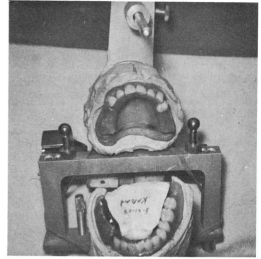

Fig. 16-2

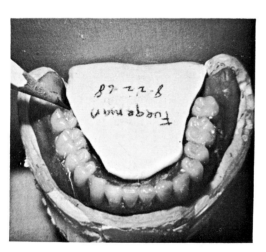

Fig. 16-3

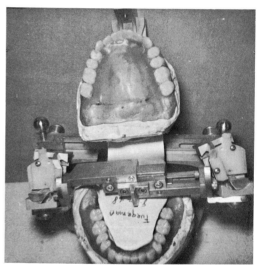

Fig. 16-4

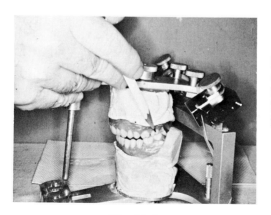

Fig. 16-5

1. After replacing the stone tongue form in the set-up (Fig. 16-1) finish the mandibular denture by setting the first and second bicuspids in a straight line toward the back, at the same height as the tongue form (Fig. 16-2).

2. Set the first and second molars by placing them in contact against the tongue form, also at the same height (Fig. 16-3).

3. Now finish the articulation by relating the upper posteriors to the lower posteriors (Fig. 16-4), and balance the occlusion to the previously made Bennett and condylar settings (Fig. 16-5). This completes the procedure.

I have found that by this method of setting the mandibular posteriors, the mandibular bicuspids and molars have a slight lingual tilt (Fig. 16-6), which adds to retention.

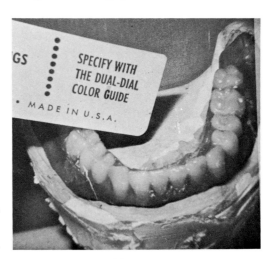

Fig. 16-6

17
Rechecking Centric Occlusion on the Try-In Denture

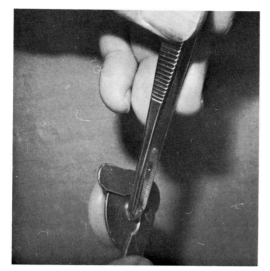

Fig. 17-1

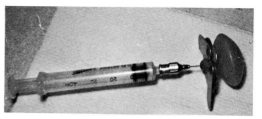

Fig. 17-2

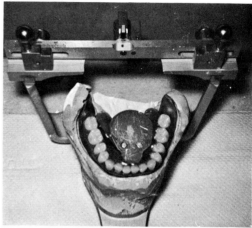

Fig. 17-4

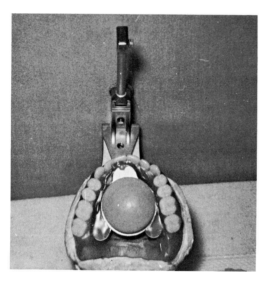

Fig. 17-3

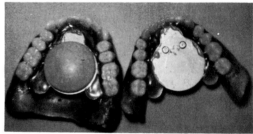

Fig. 17-5

After the upper and lower dentures have had the air bubble apparatus[1] (air centric recheck apparatus) inserted between them, centric occlusion is rechecked in the following manner.

1. Work the air cushion through the hole in the upper platform by pulling it with tweezers (Fig. 17-1).

[1] Air centric recheck apparatus. Modern Denture Research Co., Box 812, Santa Monica, Cal. 90406

2. Inflate the air cushion by injecting air by syringe through the rubber tip, which, incidentally, is self-sealing (Fig. 17-2).

3. Attach the upper platform to the palate of the maxillary try-in below the teeth (Fig. 17-3) by means of sticky wax.

4. Attach the lower platform to the mandibular denture just below the occlusal and incisal tips of the teeth by means of wax (Fig. 17-4).

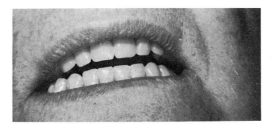

Fig. 17–6

5. Place these try-in dentures with the attached appartaus (Fig. 17–5) in the patient's mouth (Fig. 17–6) and have him practice sliding the dentures lightly back and forth (into protrusive and retrusive position) against the interposed air bubble. It is always a good idea to place your thumb on the patient's chin when he achieves a retrusive position to make sure the mandible returns all the way back posteriorly to home base. I must caution again that when checking centric position it is always necessary to check for muscle spasms. If present, they must be eliminated (as described in Chapter 6).

6. After practicing with the patient to retrude the mandible to home base (all the way back), we now are ready to recheck centric by the use of a zinc oxide Eugenol cement.[1]

7. Place petrolatum on the occlusal and incisal areas of the maxillary teeth.

8. Squeeze on a mixing pad equal parts of the base and accelerator components of Temp-Bond material (Fig. 17–7).

9. To accelerate the setting time, add a small dot of water to the spatula (Fig. 17–8).

10. Spatulate the two materials for about 10 seconds.

11. Place a small amount of this mixture in three places on the lower denture—in the molar regions on both sides and in the incisal area of the two centrals (Fig. 17–9).

[1] Temp-Bond, Kerr Mfg. Co., Detroit, Mich.

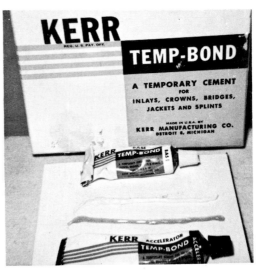

Fig. 17–7

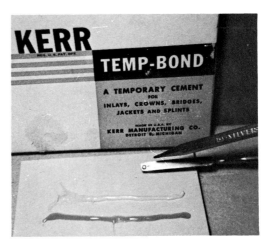

Fig. 17–8

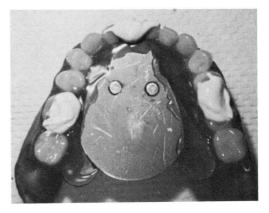

Fig. 17–9

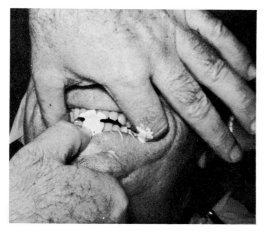

Fig. 17-10

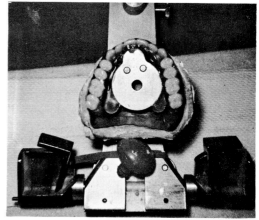

Fig. 17-11

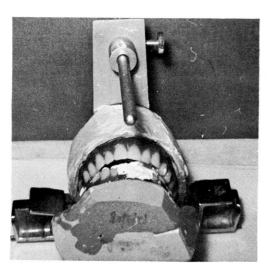

Fig. 17-12

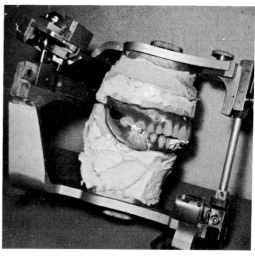

Fig. 17-13

12. Insert the lower denture into the mouth—retrude the mandible and have the patient close and hold under pressure in centric occlusion until the Temp-Bond cement has set (Fig. 17-10). With practice you can control this setting time so that the material will set within 30 seconds. (The teeth of the two dentures must not contact.)

13. When set, remove the dentures from the mouth.

14. Place the upper try-in denture on the articulated model (Fig. 17-11), but first remove the air cushion.

15. Reattach the lower Temp-Bond centric recording (Fig. 17-12). But first remove the previously articulated mandibular model from the articulator.

16. Finish the articulation (Fig. 17-13).

17. Recheck the Bennett movements and condylar inclinations recorded previously.

18

Providing for Bennett Movement and Condylar Inclinations on the Set-Up

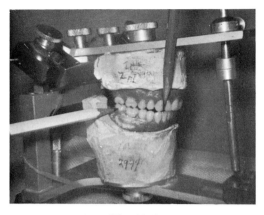

Fig. 18-1

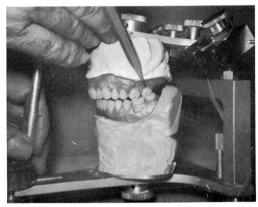

Fig. 18-2

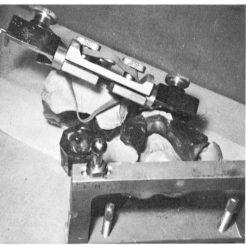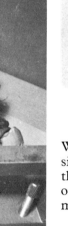

Fig. 18-3

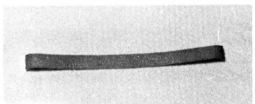

Fig. 18-4

We now provide for a "balanced" occlusion by insuring that there is contact at three points when the teeth are in eccentric occlusion. This is done in the following manner.

1. Move the articulator to one side and make sure that on the working side of the dentition (Fig. 18-1) there is contact on the cuspid and first or second molar, while on the balancing side, contact on the first molars (Fig. 18-2).

2. For balancing the opposite side of the dentition, repeat Step 1 making sure that there is two-point contact on the working side and one-point contact on the balancing side.

PLACING THE RUBBERBAND ON THE WHIP MIX ARTICULATOR

1. Separate the two parts of the articulator (Fig. 18-3).

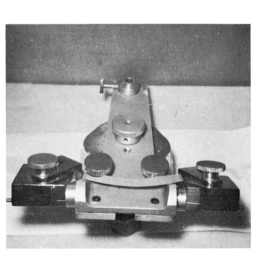

Fig. 18-5

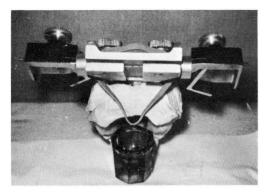

Fig. 18-6

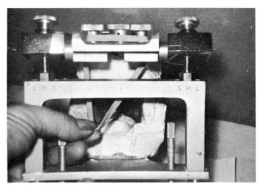

Fig. 18-7

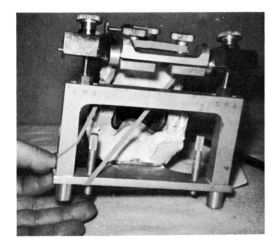

Fig. 18-8

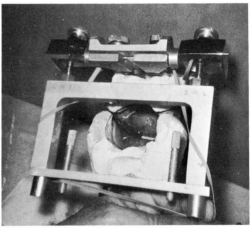

Fig. 18-9

2. Bring a No. 64^{13}/$_{16}$ oz. rubberband (Fig. 18-4) around the top part of the articulator so that it hooks in front of both condyle screws (as you look at the back of the instrument) (Fig. 18-5), with its bottom part hanging loose (Fig. 18-6).

3. Put the two parts of the articulator together (Fig. 18-7), grasping the rubberband with one hand, hook it around one of the legs (Fig. 18-8) of the lower part of the instrument.

4. Once you have engaged one leg, grasp the band on the opposite side and hook it around the other leg (Fig. 18-9). The band now holds the instrument in place (Fig. 18-10).

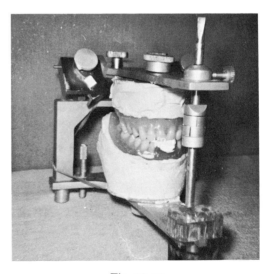

Fig. 18-10

19

Characterization of the Buccal, Lingual and Palatal Aspects of Wax Try-Ins

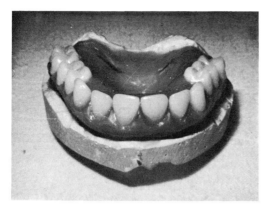

Fig. 19–1

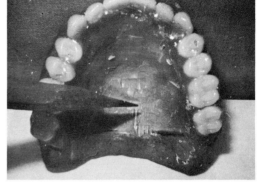

Fig. 19–2

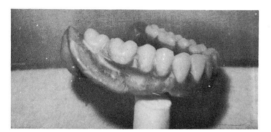

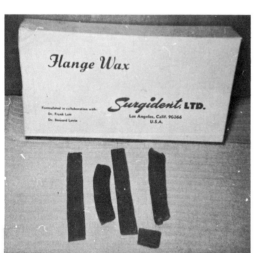

Fig. 19–3

Fig. 19–4

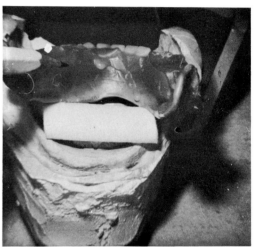

Fig. 19–5

After the wax cases have been balanced to permit proper Bennett movement and condylar inclinations, they are removed from the articulator. The next step involves contouring the waxed surfaces to reproduce natural tissue structures.

1. On the upper wax try-in, scoop out the red wax on the buccal surface from a point distal to the cuspid all the way back to the buccal tuberosity. This is done on both the right and left sides of the denture (Fig. 19–1).

2. Scoop out the wax on the entire lingual aspect near the teeth and thin out slightly the wax on the palatal section that accommodates the tongue (Fig. 19–2).

3. On the lower wax try-in, scoop out the wax on the buccal surface from a point distal to the cuspid all the way back past the second molar (Fig. 19–3).

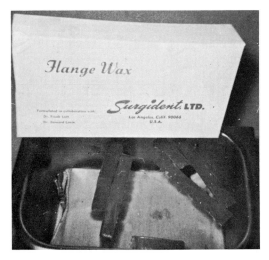

Fig. 19-6

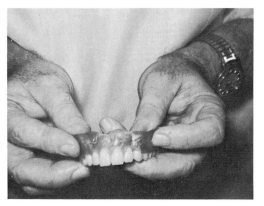

Fig. 19-7

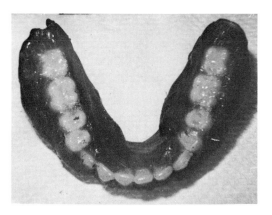

Fig. 19-8

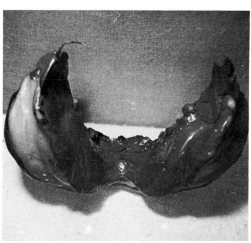

Fig. 19-9

4. Scoop out the wax on the entire lingual aspect on the lower try-in[1] (Fig. 19-4).

5. Cut strips of flange wax (Fig. 19-5) and place them in a Hanau heater in water heated to 110°F (Fig. 19-6).

6. After the wax strips have been heated for 5 minutes, remove them as needed and mold them with your fingers around the scooped out areas on the buccal surface of the upper try-in (Fig. 19-7).

7. Slightly heat this wax with an alcohol torch and place the denture in the patient's mouth.

8. Place more wax from the heated water around the scooped out areas on the buccal and lingual aspects (Fig. 19-8) of the lower try-in denture (Fig. 19-9).

9. As in Step 7, slightly heat this wax with an alcohol torch and place it in the patient's mouth.

10. Instruct him to bring the upper and lower teeth into occlusion and to perform

[1] Rubber base material instead of wax may be used for the characterization of the lingual surface of the mandibular denture.

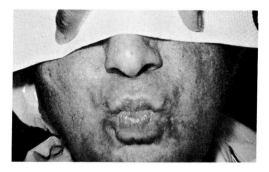

Fig. 19–10

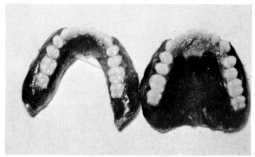

Fig. 19–11

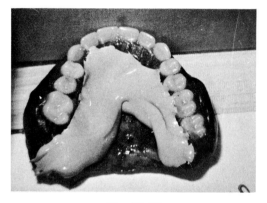

Fig. 19–12

mouth gymnastics, including the motions of sucking and swallowing (Fig. 19–10).

11. While the patient is doing this, ask him to press now and again the tip of his tongue against the lingual surfaces of the mandibular anterior teeth.

12. After two minutes of sucking and swallowing, remove the try-in dentures (Fig. 19–11) from the mouth and, using loops, examine for excessive or insufficient wax. If too much wax was used, it will work itself over and between the teeth; if too little, it will look dull and be absent in some areas. When in doubt, it is always better to have an excess of wax because it can be cut off later.

13. Complete the characterization by compensating for the excessive or insufficient amounts of wax.

We now turn our attention to the characterization of the palate.[1]

14. Replace the characterized mandibular try-in denture in the patient's mouth.

15. Place petrolatum upon the labial, buccal and occlusal surfaces of the teeth as well as the characterized wax surfaces of both dentures. This precaution prevents any excess rubber base (to be used in Step 16) from adhering to these surfaces, causing distortion upon removal from the mouth.

---

[1] Most of us have heard patients remark after we have inserted full upper and lower dentures and they have eaten several meals, "Doctor, since you placed these dentures in my mouth, the part covering the roof of my mouth has made me lose my taste sensation." Our answer to these patients usually is: "Don't be concerned. You get your sense of taste from taste buds in your tongue and not from the roof of your mouth. In a short time your mouth will adjust and taste sensation will return." This explanation is somewhat erroneous. Although it is true that taste sensation comes primarily from the taste buds in the tongue and not from the roof of the mouth, the tongue contacting the upper denture during swallowing does affect one's sense of taste. Many patients when they swallow have a space between their tongue and the denture roof, called the space of Donders. If it is not eliminated and as a result the patient's tongue does not contact the palate, he experiences a lack of taste sensation. This characteristic was brought out many years ago by investigators, foremost among whom was Dr. M.M. DeVan. Thus, it is important to eliminate the reason for the patient's complaint of lack of taste. This is accomplished during the procedure described in Steps 14 through 18.

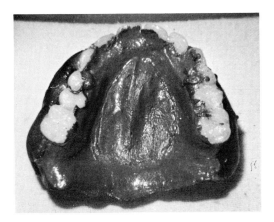

Fig. 19-13

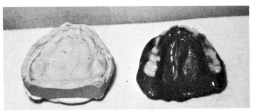

Fig. 19-14

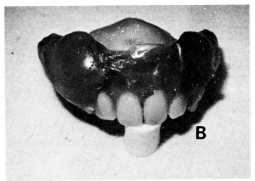

Fig. 19-15B

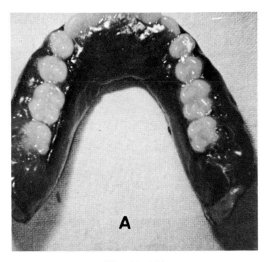

Fig. 19-15A

16. Mix equal parts of a white and brown rubber base impression material (Neo-Plex or Static-X) and place it on the palatal aspect of the upper try-in denture in a horseshoe configuration slightly below the gingival margins of the teeth (Fig. 19-12).

17. Place the upper try-in denture in the patient's mouth and instruct him to bring the teeth together in occlusion.

18. Have him place the tip of his tongue against the lingual surfaces of the upper teeth, swallow hard, and hold the swallow for 10 seconds or so. Have him repeat this

three times, with the teeth in contact. At the end of this procedure, the rubber base —partly set by this time—will have been distributed over the surface of the palate, which will have eliminated the space of Donders (Fig. 19-13).

Characterization of the dentures in the manner described (Figs. 19-14 and 19-15) gives a true representation of the lingual and palatal surfaces, and if the rest of the technic is followed carefully, the tongue and cheeks will be a tremendous aid in the retention of the dentures during function. Besides aiding in retention, such characterization gives the correct anatomic fullness to the face, which is physiologically of great importance.

I must caution that during the construction of the dentures we must continually emphasize our objectives to the patient. Tell him that the dentures will be, look, and feel quite thick, but that this is what his mouth requires for satisfactory and comfortable function.

20
Record of Face-Bow Transfer

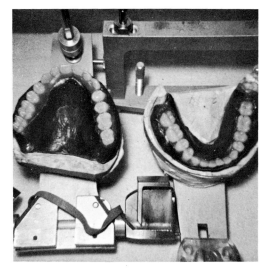

Fig. 20-1

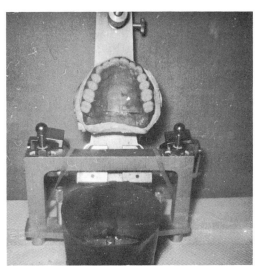

Fig. 20-2

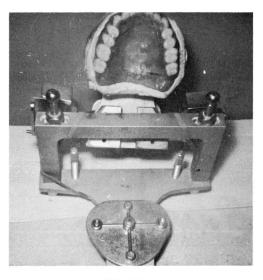

Fig. 20-3

Fig. 20-4

1. The characterized try-in dentures are now returned to the models on the articulator (Fig. 20-1). If the characterized wax has gone slightly beyond the peripheries, the case might not seat on the models. Since we do not need it, cut that portion of the wax away in order to permit the seating of the case on the models.

2. Remove the lower try-in denture, model, and ring from the articulator (Fig. 20-2).

3. Place a new ring on the lower platform of the articulator (Fig. 20-3).

4. Place a sheet of red wax around this lower ring so that it will hold poured stone (Fig. 20-4).

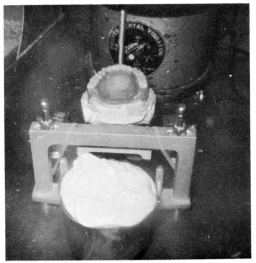

Fig. 20–5

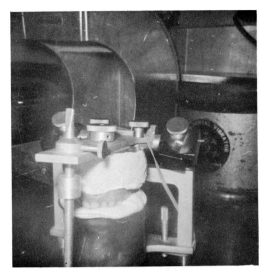

Fig. 20–6

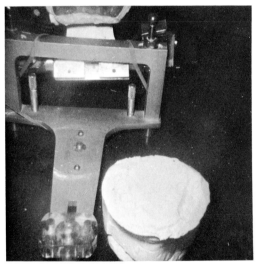

Fig. 20–7

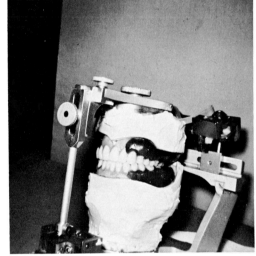

Fig. 20–8

5. Thoroughly spread petrolatum on the occlusal and incisal surfaces of the maxillary teeth.

6. Mix fast-set stone and pour it into the lower trough (Fig. 20–5).

7. Lower the upper part of the articulator which holds the upper try-in denture until the occlusal and incisal edges of the teeth indent the stone mass to about 1 to 1.5 mm. (Fig. 20–6).

8. When the stone index has set, open the articulator and remove this lower face-bow record for future use (Fig. 20–7).

9. Replace the lower try-in denture, model, and ring on the articulator (Fig. 20–8). Make sure that the teeth have not moved out of position.

21

Removal of Dentures from the Articulator and their Dispatch to the Laboratory

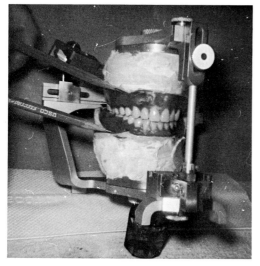

Fig. 21-1

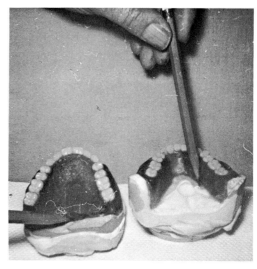

Fig. 21-2

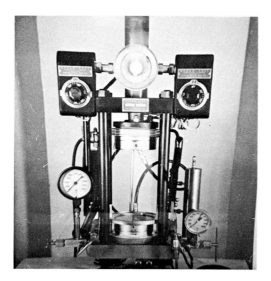

Fig. 21-3

1. Wax the cases to the stone models with red wax (Fig. 21-1).

2. Remove the cases from the articulator (Fig. 21-2) and give them to the laboratory technician with instructions (a) to duplicate the outside as well as the insides of the dentures, (b) to do very little finishing or polishing of the exterior surfaces, and (c) to leave the peripheral areas unaltered.[1]

---

[1] During the past 10 years I have used the Hydro-Cast processor (Fig. 21-3) (Kay-See Dental Mfg. Co., Kansas City, Mo.) finding that dentures thus processed fit much better than those made by any method previously tried by me. The major advantages are: a denser-finished case (no porosity), no visible shrinking away from the model, no movement of teeth, no open bite, and a more accurate duplication from the final impression. Disadvantages of the technic are that the equipment is expensive, the technician must be willing to accept instruction on how to operate the equipment and to pay attention to fine detail, and the method is more expensive to the extent that it requires more time than some others. Nonetheless, the advantages are many and important, far outweighing the disadvantages noted.

22

Return of Finished Dentures from the Laboratory with Remount Models

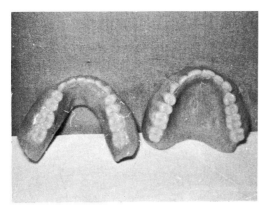

Fig. 22-1

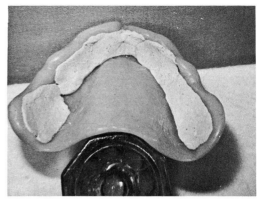

Fig. 22-2

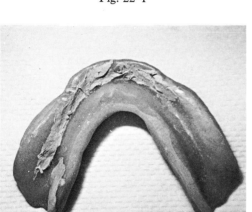

Fig. 22-3

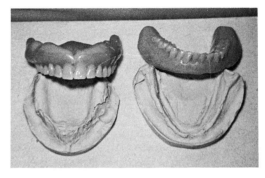

Fig. 22-4

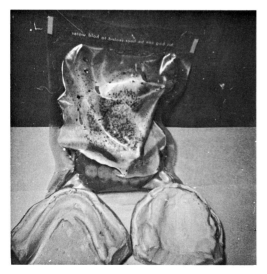

Fig. 22-5

1. Instruct the laboratory technician that after he finishes the dentures he is to relieve the undercuts with plastercine or soft paper and pour remount models.

2. Also, explain to the technician that before or after he finishes the full upper and lower dentures (Fig. 22-1) he is to make these remount models in the following manner.

    a. Place plastercine or any soft wax into any of the slight undercuts of the upper denture (Fig. 22-2) and the lower denture (Fig. 22-3).

    b. Make plaster cast models of the upper and lower dentures.

    c. When the plaster sets, separate these casts from the dentures (Fig. 22-4).

    d. Seal the dentures in a water container (Fig. 22-5) and return the dentures and the remount models to the dentist.

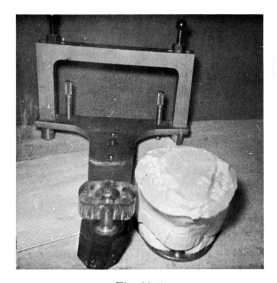

Fig. 22-6

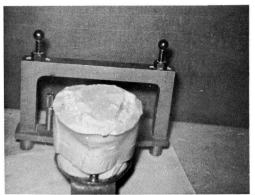

Fig. 22-7

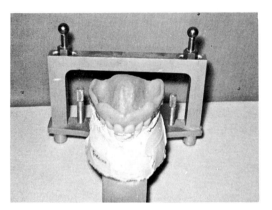

Fig. 22-8

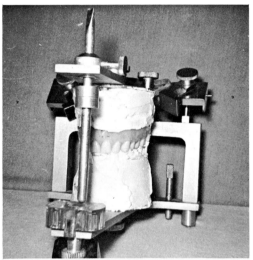

Fig. 22-9

3. Upon receiving the dentures and re-mount models from the technician, replace the remount plaster jig (Fig. 22-6) on the lower part of the articulator (Fig. 22-7).

4. Place the upper denture on the remount cast into this jig (Fig. 22-8) and place the upper remount plaster model into the denture.

5. With plaster, articulate this upper cast to the upper part of the articulator (Fig. 22-9).

6. Remove the lower remount plaster jig (Fig. 22-10).

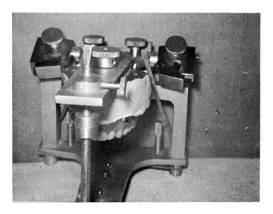

Fig. 22-10

23
Insertion of the Diagnostic Air Bubble in the Finished Dentures

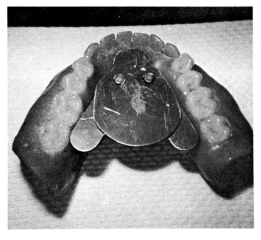

Fig. 23-1

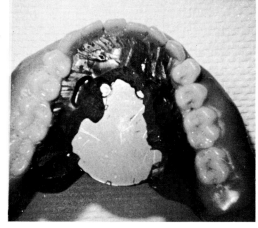

Fig. 23-2

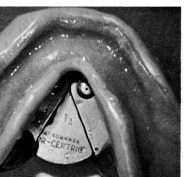

Fig. 23-3

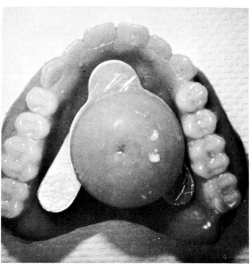

Fig. 23-4

Because in denture fabrication it is necessary to use a stone composition, wax, shellac trays, etc., and because we realize that these materials cause contractions and expansions, which may have altered the balance of our teeth, it is a must to recheck the occlusion of the teeth on these dentures. This is accomplished, using the diagnostic air bubble, in the following manner.

1. Place the lower platform of the diagnostic air bubble on the lower denture lingual surface just a few millimeters below the occlusal surfaces of the teeth (Fig. 23-1).

2. Secure this platform to the denture by means of sticky wax or compound placed on both areas—occlusally (Fig. 23-2) and underneath—lingually (Fig. 23-3).

3. Now place the inflated bubble unit of the diagnostic apparatus into the palatal

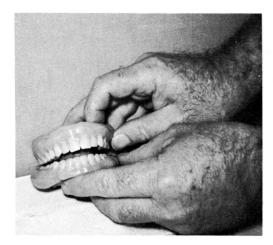

Fig. 23-5

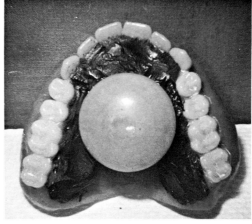

Fig. 23-6

portion of the upper denture (Fig. 23-4), making sure that the bubble is inflated sufficiently so that when in contact with the platform on the lower denture, the distance between the virtually occluding upper and lower dentures is 3 to 4 mm. (Fig. 23-5).

4. Secure the bubble apparatus to the denture by means of sticky wax or compound (Fig. 23-6).

24
Verifying Centric Occlusion on the Finished Dentures

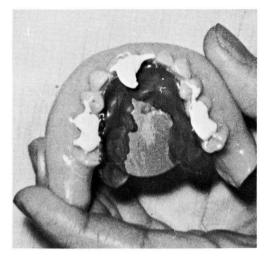

Fig. 24–1

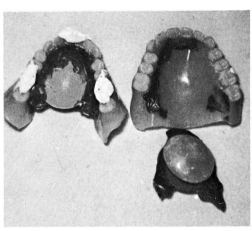

Fig. 24–2

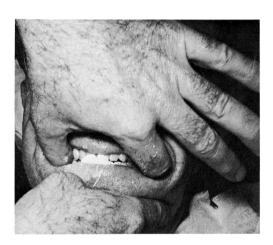

Fig. 24–3

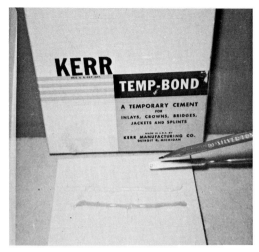

Fig. 24–4

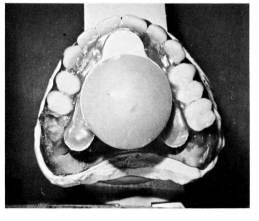

Fig. 24–5

Since the Bennett movements, condylar inclinations, recordings and face-bow records were preserved, it is only necessary to recheck the centric occlusion. This is accomplished in the following manner.

1. Spread petrolatum upon the occlusal and incisal surfaces of the upper denture only, and insert this upper denture into the patient's mouth.

2. Prepare a mixture of Temp-Bond according to the directions provided, and

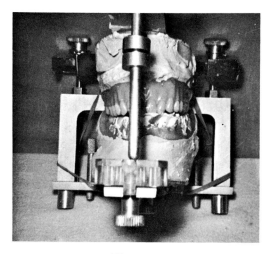

Fig. 24–6

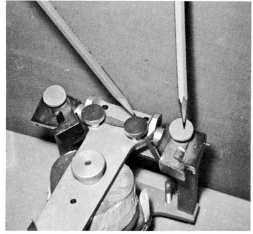

Fig. 24–7

add to this a small drop of water while it is being spatulated (Fig. 24–1).

3. After spatulating for no more than 6 to 8 seconds, place three small mounds of the mixture in the area of the first molar and of the second bicuspid, and on the anterior teeth of the lower denture (Fig. 24–2), and immediately place in the patient's mouth on the lower ridge.

4. After retruding the patient's lower jaw to centric position, have him close, and hold his jaw in centric position until the Temp-Bond sets (Fig. 24–3). When properly mixed with a drop of water, Temp-Bond will set within 20 to 30 seconds.

5. When the mixture has set, remove the dentures from the patient's mouth (Fig. 24–4). The bubble on the upper denture

may be removed now or as the next step. The removal of the bubble permits the securing of the upper against the lower without springing away from the teeth.

6. Place the upper denture (Fig. 24–5) on the upper articulated remount model.

7. Position the lower denture, held at three points with Temp-Bond to the upper denture.

8. After securing the two dentures together with hard red wax, fit the lower remount model in place and finish the articulation on the instrument (Fig. 24–6).

9. Recheck the articulator to make sure it is set for the correct Bennett movements and condylar inclinations (Fig. 24–7).

25

Adjusting the Occlusion of Finished Dentures on the Articulator

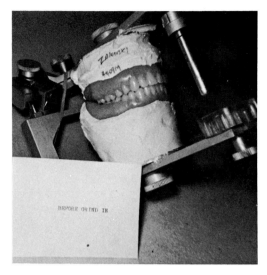

Fig. 25-1

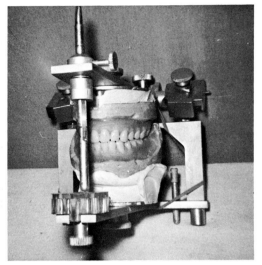

Fig. 25-2

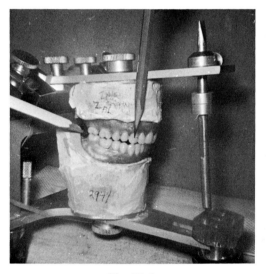

Fig. 25-3

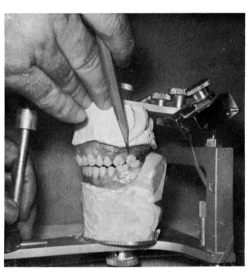

Fig. 25-4

1. Begin by checking for prematurities in centric occlusion (Fig. 25-1).

2. Grind away interferences in such a manner that you achieve the same interdigitation of the molars and bicuspids that you had with the adjusted wax try-in dentures (Fig. 25-2).

3. Next check left lateral movement. Move the articulator to the left in such a way that the right buccal cusp surfaces of the maxillary molars contact the right buccal cusp surfaces of the mandibular molars (Fig. 25-3), and also the opposing cuspids contact on the same side.

4. While the instrument is in this position, check the left side (the balancing side) to make sure that the lingual cusps of the maxillary second molar contacts the buccal cusps of the mandibular second molar (Fig. 25-4).

5. Because I believe that there should be bilateral balance in full denture prosthesis, I keep adjusting the left lateral eccentric occlusion (which, in a check bite technique, and following the Whip Mix instructions, actually combines Bennett movement and condylar inclination) until the working side shows contact on the buccal aspect of the upper and lower molars and the upper and lower cuspids, and the balancing side shows contact between the lingual aspect of the upper second molar and the buccal aspect of the lower second molar.

6. To adjust the other lateral occlusion, the articulator is moved to the right and Steps 3, 4, and 5 are repeated for two-point contact on the working side and one-point contact on the balancing side.

7. Recheck the case for balances in centric and eccentric occlusion.

26

The Need For Tissue Treatment

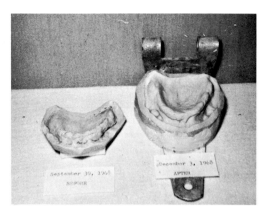

Fig. 26–1

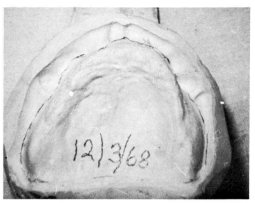

Fig. 26–2

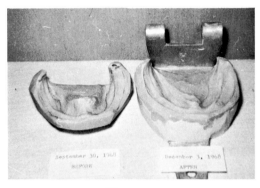

Fig. 26–3

All full upper and lower dentures should be fitted with due consideration of the dynamic movements that occur when the wearer actually uses the dentures during talking, chewing and deglutition. Since the original impressions were taken under more or less static conditions (with the least amount of compression), in order to allow for dynamic conditions it is necessary to place tissue treatment under the finished dentures and, following the completion of the treatment process, make these modified dentures permanent.[1]

When the patient has firm, well-defined, non-resilient and nonpathologic tissue, dentures can be constructed without tissue treatment. However, where the tissues have suffered abuse owing to previous dentures that were ill-fitting for one reason or another (as in a closed or open vertical), tissue treatment is imperative.

[1] As described in Chapter 29.

Although it is often said that "tissue contained in the denture cannot go anywhere," I believe that displaced and misshaped tissue, when covered by a denture and subjected to the dynamic stress of daily use, reacts like a sausage-shaped carnival balloon—when pressed on one end, it changes shape. Furthermore, after treating such tissue and comparing the progress models of the jaws from treatment stage to treatment stage, we see that it is not only feasible but essential to return these mouths to normal (Fig. 26–1). If not, the patient may never be comfortable. In many of these cases, comparison photographs of the final treated case and the original (Fig. 26–2) shows tissue that appears not to have come from the same mouth.

Let me stress, however, that tissue treatment alone, without sound principles having been applied first in the construction of the dentures, can do more harm than good.

The patient under treatment should be seen for a change of treatment every 3 days. The length of tissue treatment depends on the condition of the tissues and its severity. The longer the patient has had ill-fitting dentures that have caused considerable displacement and tissue hypertrophy, the longer the tissue treatment will take. Cases that are not too severe can be finished (tissue treated) within 2 to 4 visits. However, I have had cases that required treatment for as long as a year and one half before the patient had complete comfort.

27

The Procedure For Tissue Treatment

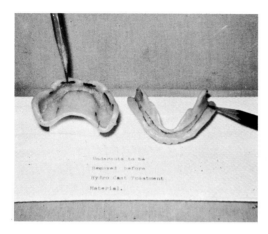

Fig. 27–1

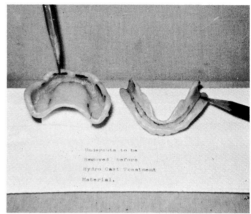

Fig. 27–2

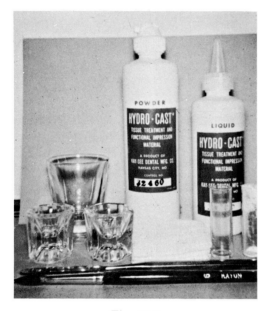

Fig. 27–3

To prepare the dentures for tissue treatment, proceed in the following manner:

1. After the upper and lower dentures have been balanced on the articulator, remove them from it and polish the occlusal and incisal surfaces.

2. Prepare the upper denture to receive the tissue treatment by removing only the slight undercuts (Fig. 27–1). Do not touch any other part of the denture.

3. Follow the same procedure when removing the undercuts (Fig. 27–2) from the lower denture. Remember, remove only the undercuts; nothing else.

The procedure for the first tissue treatment is as follows:

1. If this is the first application of tissue treatment to the dentures, do one denture at a time. Place the prepared lower denture (with the undercuts removed) into the mouth.

2. Mix the tissue treatment[1] (Fig. 27–3) in proportions of 1 part liquid to 1¼ parts powder.

3. Pour the liquid into the container first and then spatulate the powder into the liquid and stir with a spatula for 10 to 15 seconds.

4. When the mixture is the consistency of heavy cream, bead with a camel's hair brush all the way around *only* the periphery of the upper denture (Fig. 27–4).

5. Place the upper beaded denture very carefully into the patient's mouth and ask

[1] Kay See Dental Mfg. Co.

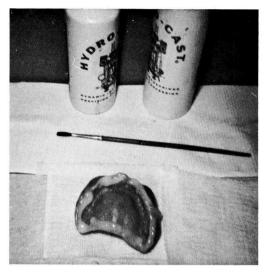

Fig. 27–4

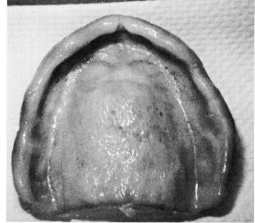

Fig. 27–5

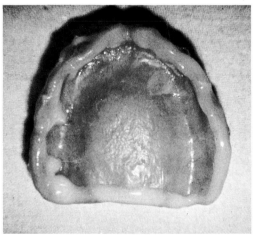

Fig. 27–6

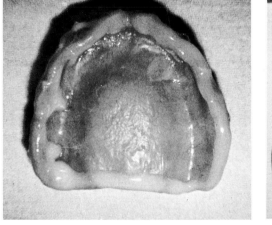

Fig. 27–7

him to bring both dentures together into contact occlusion.

6. While the dentures are being held lightly together in occlusion, instruct the patient to go through mouth gymnastics, which consist of puckering, grinning, sucking and swallowing. Have him continue these gymnastics for 3 minutes.

7. After 3 minutes of gymnastics, have the patient talk for three minutes. Mouth gymnastics and talking cause the tissue

treatment under function to be sucked into, and between, the upper denture and the underlying tissues without upsetting the occlusion.

8. Remove the upper denture and examine for tissue treatment deficiencies over the denture (Fig. 27–5).

9. After drying with an air syringe this partially treated upper denture, make a new mix of tissue treatment material, this time 1 to 1, and apply over the entire peri-

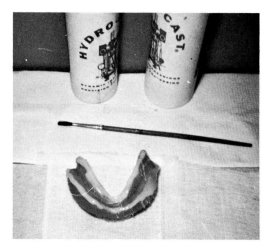

Fig. 27–8

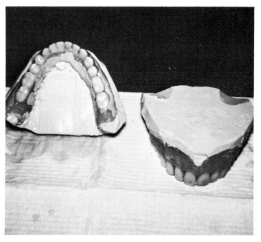

Fig. 27–9

phery (Fig. 27-6) and over the previous beaded material in a much thinner consistency.

10. Re-insert the upper denture into the mouth and have the patient repeat Steps 5 through 8.

11. Following these two paintings with tissue treatment, we usually find that the entire denture is now completely covered (Fig. 27-7). However, if a few spots have been missed in the palatal region, lightly paint over such areas with a fresh 1-to-1 mix, re-insert the dentures into the mouth, and have the patient hold in occlusion for 6 minutes.

12. When the upper denture is satisfactory, remove both dentures from the mouth and trim off any excess material from their occlusal and incisal areas.

13. Replace the tissue-treated upper denture in the patient's mouth.

14. After air drying the lower denture, proceed to treat it in the same manner as was done in Steps 2 through 11 for the upper denture. A lower denture with a

completely covered periphery is shown in Figure 27-8.

15. Dismiss the patient with instructions to attempt to eat regular meals, to sleep with the dentures in place. They should be removed only to be washed, in cold tap water, and replaced in the mouth immediately. The patient should be scheduled for a return in 3 days for a change of treatment.

The procedure for the second application of tissue treatment is as follows:

1. When the patient returns in 3 days, ask him about the efficiency and comfort of his dentures. He is usually very enthusiastic. Remove the dentures from the mouth, air dry, and examine them for denuded areas. If a great deal of the bearing area over the ridges is denuded, the vertical is open. Thus, we recognize that tissue treatment, in addition to its other advantages, is a check on vertical dimension.

2. Mark the denuded areas with an indelible pencil. These tissue-treated dentures are now handled the same as wash impressions.

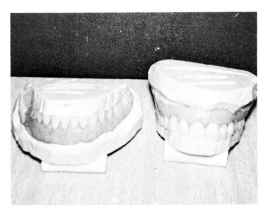

Fig. 27–10

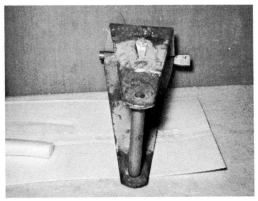

Fig. 27–11

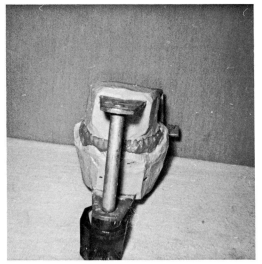

Fig. 27–12

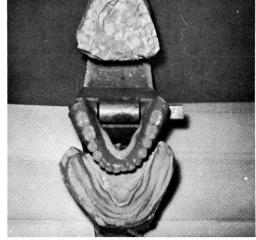

Fig. 27–13

3. Pour stone models (Fig. 27–9).

4. Make occlusal and incisal indices (Fig. 27–10).

5. A jig[1] (Fig. 27–11) is now used like a hinge articulator, having an anterior pin to maintain the vertical. Articulate each denture separately using a separate jig for each (Fig. 27–12).

[1] The use of the jig during tissue treatment has the double purpose of permitting us to replace the dentures each time in the same position in the mouth during treatments, and allowing us to delegate to auxiliary personnel the removal of the old material and its replacement.

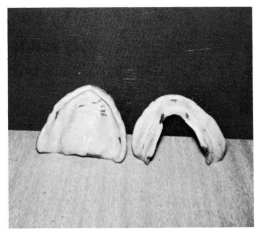

Fig. 27–14

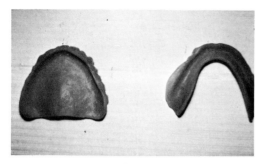

Fig. 27–15

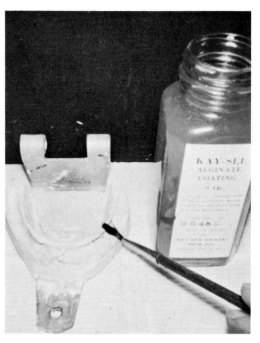

Fig. 27–16

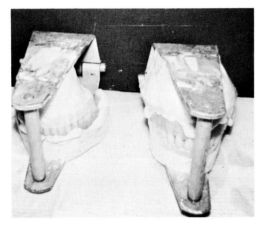

Fig. 27–17

6. When the plaster has set, separate each jig (Fig. 27–13).

7. Using a No. 12 round bur, first remove the acrylic over the areas marked with indelible pencil (Fig. 27–14).

8. Using burs and a scraper, remove the remainder of the old tissue treatment (Fig. 27–15), exposing the entire inside of the denture.

9. With a special liquid separator (Kay See Dental Mfg. Co.) paint the denture models (Fig. 27–16).

10. Mix 1 part tissue treatment liquid to 1¼ part tissue treatment powder and spatulate for 20 to 30 seconds.

11. When mixture is the consistency of sour cream, place the treatment into each denture, position on the model, and close the jig (Fig. 27–17).

12. Place elastic bands around the jig to keep it together (Fig. 27–18).

13. Place in a pan of warm water for 5 minutes. If 5 or 6 drops of a wetting agent (Fig. 27–19) (Kay See Dental Mfg. Co.) is added to the pan, it helps to break the surface tension of the sticky tissue treatment. It also prevents the material from sticking to the fingers and knife when the excess is trimmed off.

14. After 5 minutes, remove from the water and trim off the excess with a knife.

15. Remove the cases from the models.

16. Prepare a 1-to-1 mixture of tissue treatment.

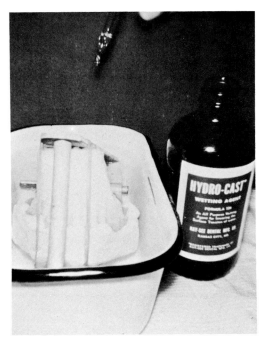

Fig. 27–18

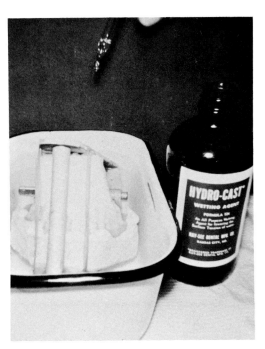

Fig. 27–19

17. While this new tissue treatment is in a thin state, paint a very light thin coating over the upper and lower denture surfaces previously treated (Fig. 27–20).

18. Insert both dentures in the mouth and have the patient hold in centric occlusion.

19. After 5 minutes, remove the dentures and cut off the slight excess while rinsing them under cold water.

20. Dismiss the patient with the same instructions as given after the first treatment —attempt to eat regular meals, sleep with the dentures in place, and remove them only to wash in cold tap water, replacing them in the mouth immediately. Have the patient return in 3 days. If these dentures are to be used as the final dentures, and you find that the tissue has made its maximum response, and if the patient is comfortable, you are ready for the final tissue treatment procedure before these dentures are finalized.

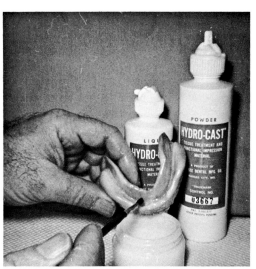

Fig. 27–20

21. Remove the dentures from the patient's mouth.

22. Thoroughly air dry the tissue-treated surfaces with an air syringe.

23. With a Q-tip paint the treated surfaces with Flo-Control (Kay See Dental Mfg. Co.) and place the dentures on the laboratory bench for 5 minutes. (Flo-Control helps to soften the old tissue treatment material.)

24. Make a new 1-to-1 mixture of tissue treatment material and apply with a brush as a bead all around and over the tissue treatment material along the peripheries of both dentures.

25. Insert both dentures in the mouth and have the patient repeat Steps 5 through 8 completed during the first tissue treatment visit.

26. If one beading is not enough, repeat the Steps 24 and 25.

27. After 6 to 8 minutes of facial gymnastics and talking, remove the dentures.

28. Trim off the excess treatment and reinsert the dentures in the patient's mouth.

29. Instruct the patient to go out and have a sandwich and a cup of coffee or tea and to return to the office in one hour.

30. When the patient returns to the office, remove the dentures from his mouth and send them to the technician for finalization, with instructions to use the Porceline procedure employed in Chapter 29.

31. When the technician returns the finalized dentures to you, repeat the procedures as described in Chapter 24.

28

Termination of Tissue Treatment

When do you stop tissue treatment? When the patient is comfortable. This means that the tissues have returned to normal and that the patient can use the denture with maximum comfort and good chewing efficiency. The length of time it takes to treat an individual case depends upon the severity of the conditions involving the oral tissue when the patient first presents for treatment.

I have found that in order to get the best results you should have the patient return to the office every three days in order to change the tissue treatment, because after three days the tissue treatment material has lost most of its working flow and not only may cause the denture to hurt the patient, but, more important, is no longer helping to restore the oral tissue to a normal state. The minimum course of tissue treatment requires four changes of tissue treatment material.

During treatment it may also be necessary to check and adjust the occlusion several times. Occlusal discrepancy may occur, especially if there were spasms of the external and internal pterygoid muscle fibre attachments of long duration, causing some rotations of the mandible. Such rotation results in a horizontal rather than an anteroposterior change in occlusion and must be corrected by rechecking with the air bubble, or, better still, with the Baptist intra-oral, extra-oral apparatus. It should be remembered that the extent of the horizontal mandibular change influences the duration of tissue treatment. However, once all the structures of the stomatognathic system return to normal—especially when the correct vertical and anteroposterior centric occlusion has been established —the tissues respond faster and the patient is comfortable with the efficient function of his dentures.

29

Duplicating the Treated Denture Bases After Final Tissue Conditioning

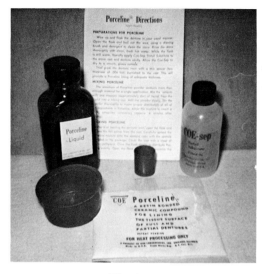

Fig. 29-1

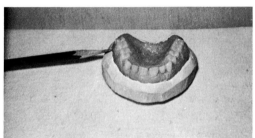

Fig. 29-2

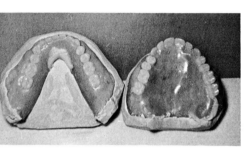

Fig. 29-3

Fig. 29-4

Two methods are satisfactory. The first involves the use of Porceline, which aids retention, and the second requires a soft reline to cushion the denture and aid retention.

THE USE OF PORCELINE

If after tissue treatment the bearing areas under the dentures do not have spinous ridges, a product called Porceline by Coe Laboratories (Fig. 29-1) can be used as a final rebase. A new plastic, it helps to reduce the surface tension on the tissue side of the denture, thereby aiding retention. This rebase-like material is applied in the following manner.

1. Remove the tissue-treated dentures (Fig. 29-2) from the patient's mouth.

2. Pour upper and lower stone models in these treated dentures (Fig. 29-3) making sure that the stone reaches to the height of the borders (Fig. 29-4) but does not extend *over* them. (This would cause the model to break when being separated from the denture.)

3. Pour stone occlusal-incisal indexes of each denture (Fig. 29-5).

4. Place the upper indexed model in a Jectron jig and mount with stone (Fig. 29-6).

5. Do the same with the lower indexed model (Fig. 29-7).

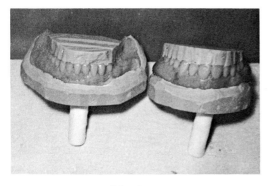

Fig. 29-5

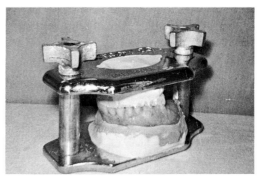

Fig. 29-6

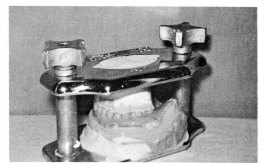

Fig. 29-7

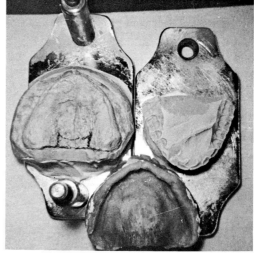

Fig. 29-8

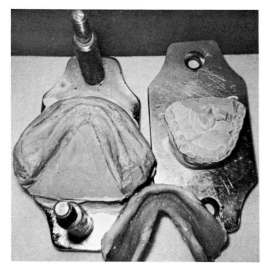

Fig. 29-9

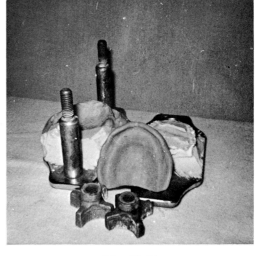

6. When stone has set, open the jigs by removing the two screw nuts (Fig. 29-8). Do the same with the lower indexed model (Fig. 29-9).

Fig. 29-10

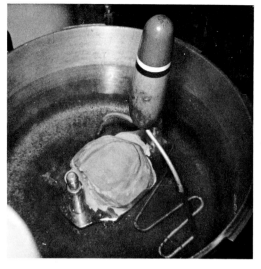

Fig. 29-11

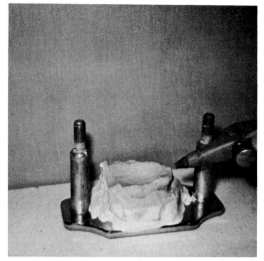

Fig. 29-12

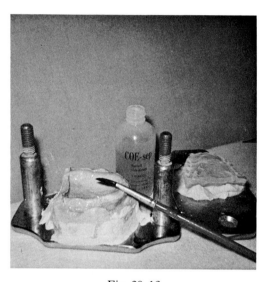

Fig. 29-13

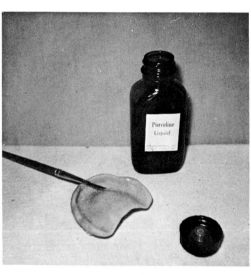

Fig. 29-14

7. Remove the impression material from the dentures (Fig. 29-10) with scrapers and Vulcanite burs.

8. Now place the models in a pressure cooker in clean water at 160° F for three minutes (Fig. 29-11).

9. Remove them from the pressure cooker, air dry with a syringe (Fig. 29-12), and paint Coe alginate separator on the warm models (Fig. 29-13).

10. Mix Porceline to the manufacturer's specifications.

11. When the Porceline reaches a doughy consistency paint the denture bases (Fig. 29-14) with Porceline liquid.

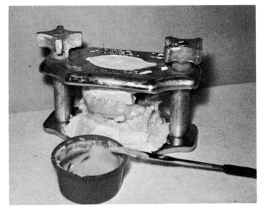

Fig. 29–15

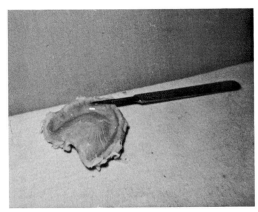

Fig. 29–16

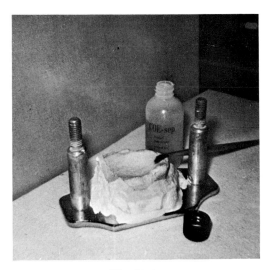

Fig. 29–17

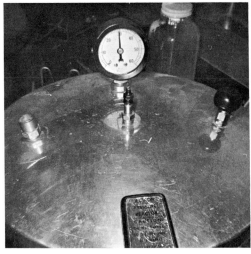

Fig. 29–18

12. Test pack with thin plastic sheets (Fig. 29–15) by closing the jig.

13. Open the jigs; if bubbles appear in the Porceline or if there is not enough, add more and test pack a second time.

14. Open the jig again and recheck as above.

15. If the results are now satisfactory trim the gross excess away (Fig. 29–16) and repaint the model with Coe alginate separator (Fig. 29–17).

16. Close the jigs, tighten the nuts and place in water in a pressure cooker at 160° F, making sure that the jigs are fully immersed.

17. Put on the cover and lock the pressure cooker (Fig. 29–18). Insert 30 lbs. of air.

18. Leave the cases to cure in the pressure cooker at 160° to 165°F for a minimum of 6 hours.

19. When the cases are cured, release the air pressure, remove the cover from the

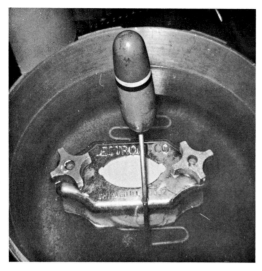

Fig. 29–19

Fig. 29–20

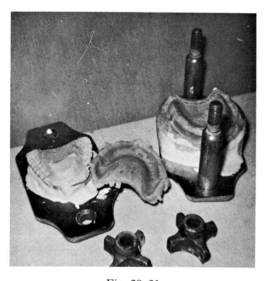

Fig. 29–21

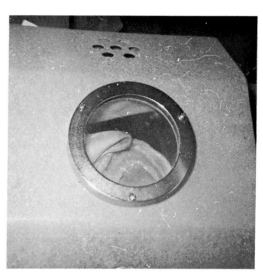

Fig. 29–22

cooker, and place the cases in cold tap water. Cool for 20 minutes (Fig. 29–19).

20. Open the jigs (Fig. 29–20) and remove the dentures from the models (Fig. 29–21).

21. Finish and polish the dentures in the usual manner.

22. Make remount models.

23. Sand blast the tissue surfaces of the dentures (Fig. 29–22), making sure that you do not handle the sand-blasted areas. This prevents contamination by the natural oils of the fingers.

24. Seal these dentures in a cellophane bag (Fig. 29–23).

25. Now proceed with the case as described in Chapters 23, 24, and 25.

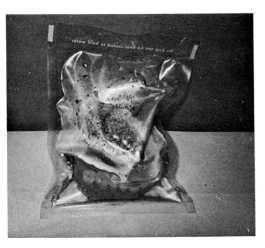

Fig. 29–23

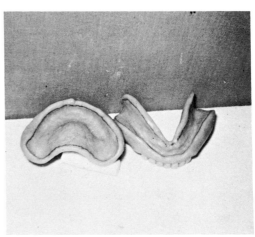

Fig. 29–24

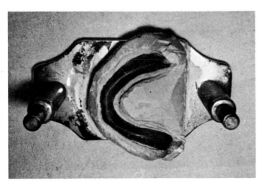

Fig. 29–25

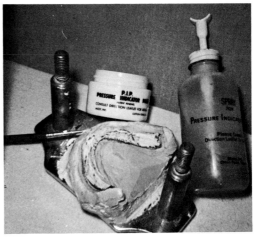

Fig. 29–26

THE USE OF A SOFT RELINE

If the upper denture reveals areas of hard bone and the lower a thin spinous ridge, a soft liner may be indicated. Of the soft liners on the market, there is one which, though not permanent, is helpful for 2 or 3 months. It is called Sofdent, and is manufactured by National Patents.[1] Although this material comes in two forms—self-cure and heat cure—I prefer the latter. It is employed in the following manner.

1. Repeat Steps 1 through 7 as employed with Porceline.

[1] Malcolm E. Boone, Indiana University School of Dentistry, was kind enough to give me the benefit of his experience and research findings on this subject. His observations on the duration of serviceability of the material agree with my own.

2. Outline with a pencil the areas upon which Sofdent is desired 2 to 3 mm. inside the peripheral borders on the dentures (Fig. 29–24). The borders must remain of hard acrylic. However, if the borders need altering we must add hard acrylic. This is done as follows.

3. Adapt one thickness of base plate wax to this outline on the models (Fig. 29–25).

4. Paint P.I.P. (Mizzy, Inc.) or some other indicator on the surface of the wax (Fig. 29–26).

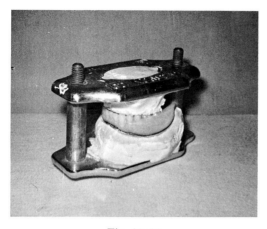

Fig. 29-27

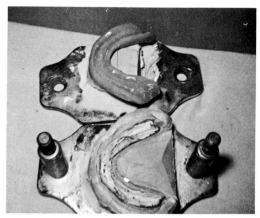

Fig. 29-28

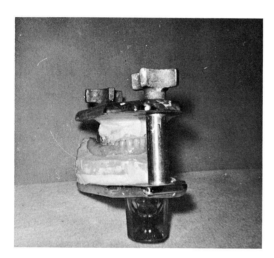

Fig. 29-29

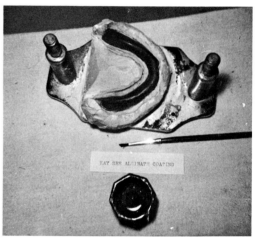

Fig. 29-30

5. Place the section of the jig that holds the denture gently in place over the model part of the jig (Fig. 29-27).

6. Reopen the jig and grind the marked areas (Fig. 29-28).

7. Repeat the above step until enough acrylic is removed to permit closing the jig (Fig. 29-29).

8. Remove P.I.P. material from the wax by wiping with carbon tetrachloride (making sure that the wax spacer remains in place).

9. Paint the model with Kay See alginate separating material (Fig. 29-30).

10. Mix Kay See "back up" acrylic. One half a unit should be enough for the average case (Fig. 29-31).

11. When the back-up material is no longer tacky, paint the inner surfaces of the denture bases with acrylic monomer (Fig. 29-32).

12. Pack the back-up acrylic into the denture bases with the wax spacer in place, making sure that there is some excess.

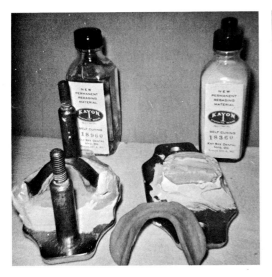

Fig. 29–31

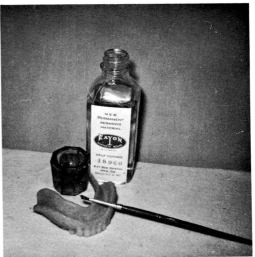

Fig. 29–32

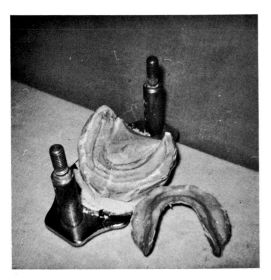

Fig. 29–33

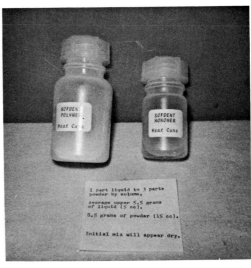

Fig. 29–34

13. Put the jigs together and tighten the nuts; place in a pressure cooker, with water at 110°F and with 30 lbs. of air pressure, and cure for 30 minutes.

14. At the end of the 30 minutes, release the air pressure, remove the cover, and cool the jigs.

15. Open the jigs (Fig. 29–33) and remove the wax spacers.

16. Prepare the heat-cured Sofdent material according to the manufacturer's direction, 5 cc. of powder to 5 cc. of liquid (Fig. 29–34). This mixture appears to be very dry until it is mixed well. (Do not add additional liquid.) Spatulate for 4 minutes

17. Paint the roughened denture base with Sofdent liquid (Fig. 29–35) and paint the model with Sofdent separator. You

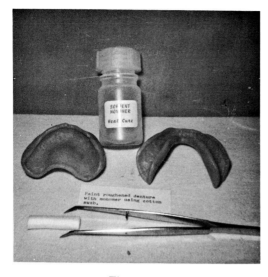

Fig. 29–35

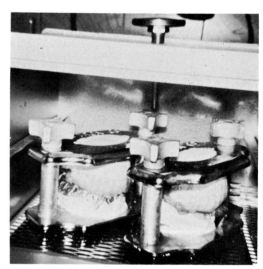

Fig. 29–36

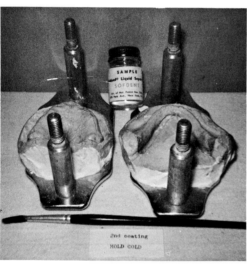

Fig. 29–37

Fig. 29–38

should paint twice; the first on the warm mold (Figs. 29–36 and 29–37).

18. Pack the material into the denture bases during the putty stage. Test pack if desired.

19. Close and tighten the nuts on the jig and place in boiling water for 2 hours in an open pot or in the Pyroplast oven (Fig. 29–38) for one hour at 175° F. However if the Pyroplast oven (Williams-Justi Co.) is used the models must be tin-foiled.

20. After boiling, remove the jigs and bench-cool for one hour.

21. When cool, trim and polish in the usual manner.

22. Since these finished dentures (Fig. 29–39 and 29–40) containing the Sofdent material have been hardened, they must be placed in water for a minimum of 24 hours

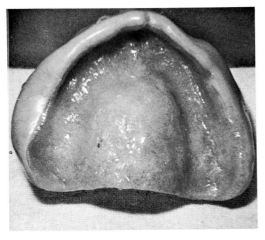

Fig. 29-39

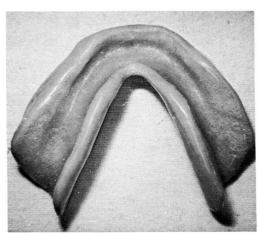

Fig. 29-40

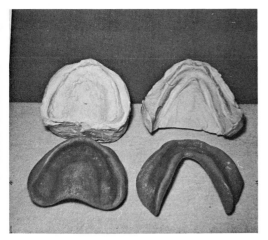

Fig. 29-41

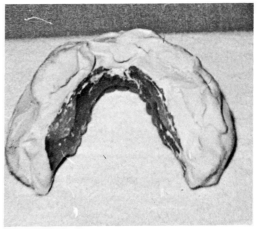

Fig. 29-42

to be fully softened. Make remount models only after you are certain that the material has fully softened (Fig. 29-41) and keep the models and the dentures in water.

23. Now repeat the procedures outlined in Chapters 23, 24 and 25.

A SOFT-CUSHIONED MATERIAL FOR TENDER, DIFFICULT-TO-FIT MOUTHS

A third material, which has been on the market for some time, if used carefully will surpass by far, I believe, the Sofdent procedure, because it lasts much longer without alteration in form or consistency. This material, called Silastic 390, by Dow Chemical, when used with the "multiple suction cup technic,"[1] preceded by the tissue treatment procedure, definitely yields gratifying results with difficult upper or lower dentures.

The procedure for lower denture is as follows.

1. After the final tissue treatment of the lower denture, remove the denture from the patient's mouth and pour stone into it (Fig. 29-42). Note that the tongue area is not covered.

[1] Jermyn, Arthur C.: J. Prost. Dent., 18:316–325, 1967 and distributed by PROKEM. Corp. 175 Norris Drive, Rochester, N. Y. 14610.

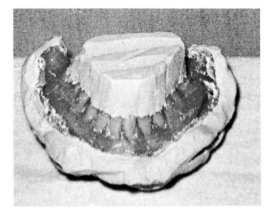

Fig. 29-43

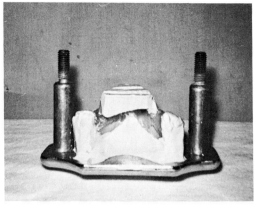

Fig. 29-44

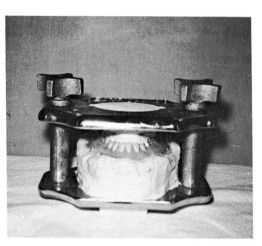

Fig. 29-45

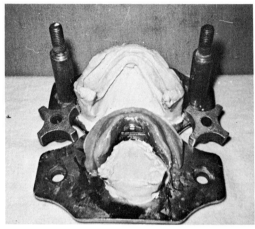

Fig. 29-46

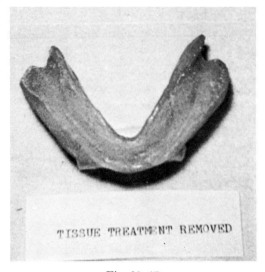

TISSUE TREATMENT REMOVED

Fig. 29-47

2. Pour an occlusal stone index model (Fig. 29-43).

3. Place the model on the jig (Fig. 29-44).

4. Lower finished mounting on the jig (Fig. 29-45).

5. Separate the jig and remove the case from the model (Fig. 29-46).

6. The tissue treatment material is removed from the periphery only about 1 mm. toward the inside of the denture and completely removed from the labial and buccal aspects (Fig. 29-47).

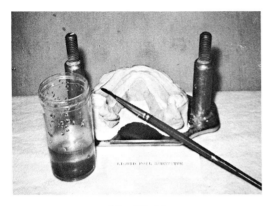

Fig. 29-48

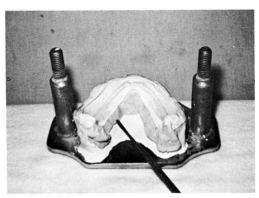

Fig. 29-49

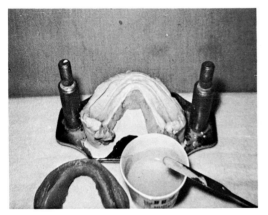

Fig. 29-50

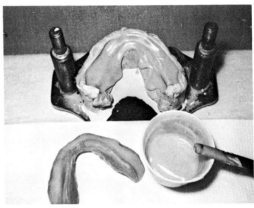

Fig. 29-51

7. Liquid foil substitute is painted on the model (Fig. 29-48).

8. Lingual undercuts beyond the model are blocked out with caulking compound (Fig. 29-49).

9. Employing the jig, the borders are now about to be added to by using a quick-cure acrylic. This acrylic[1] must be fluid and of a smooth consistency (Fig. 29-50).

10. This acrylic is now spread on the model and over the entire inside of the tissue-treated denture (Fig. 29-51). (Since this acrylic is smooth-flowing, it will not

[1] Acribase, Jectron Co., Howmet Corp., Chicago, Ill.

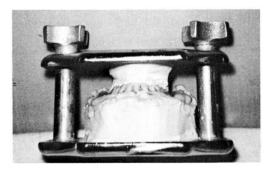

Fig. 29-52

raise the bite and will be squeezed away from the tissue-treated sections of the denture.)

11. The denture is now placed on the model; the jig is closed and securely bolted (Fig. 29-52).

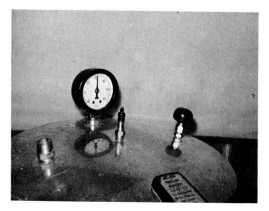

Fig. 29–53

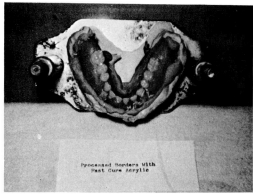

Fig. 29–54

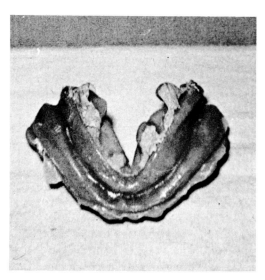

Fig. 29–55

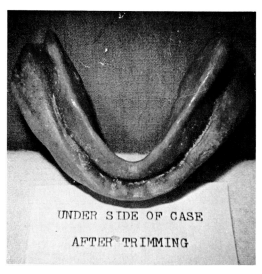

Fig. 29–56

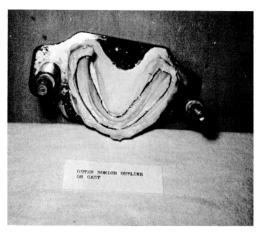

Fig. 29–57

12. The jig is now placed in the pressure cooker. Warm water is added and the lid is closed; 30 lbs. of air pressure is introduced, and the case is left in cooker to process for 20 minutes (Fig. 29–53).

13. After 20 minutes the air in the pressure cooker is released and the jig is opened, exposing the processed borders (Fig. 29–54).

14. The denture removed from the model shows new acrylic excess over the borders, before trimming (Fig. 29–55).

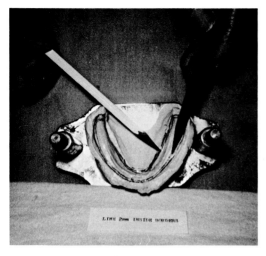

Fig. 29-58

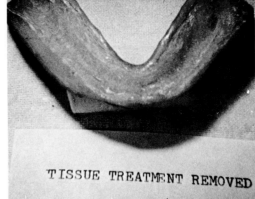

Fig. 29-59

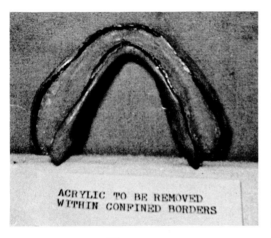

Fig. 29-60

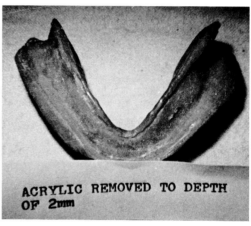

Fig. 29-61

15. The denture borders are trimmed (Fig. 29-56).

16. The borders are outlined on the cast with a soft pencil (Fig. 29-57).

17. Parallel lines are drawn all the way around the buccal and lingual surfaces of the cast 2 mm. from the original border outline and towards the center of the ridge (Fig. 29-58).

At this juncture, palpate the mouth for any hard areas on the ridge and mark them on the model.

18. The remainder of the tissue treatment is removed from the denture (Fig. 29-59).

19. A line is drawn all the way around the inside of the denture about 1 mm. below the periphery (Fig. 29-60).

20. Within the confines of the border line, to a depth of about 2 mm., remove acrylic from the inside of the denture with a large round bur (Fig. 29-61). (This acrylic border edge should be made so that the junction of the hard acrylic and soft reline

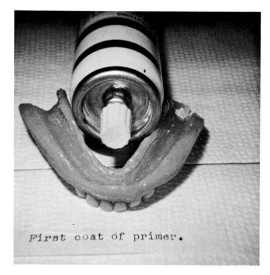

First coat of primer.

Fig. 29–62

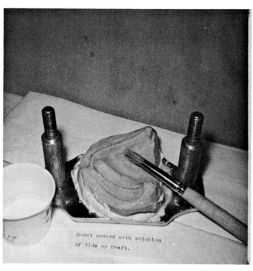

Second coat of primer.

Fig. 29–63

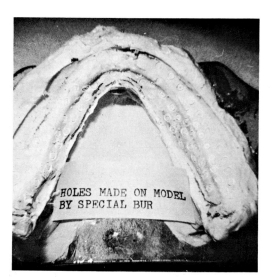

HOLES MADE ON MODEL
BY SPECIAL BUR

Fig. 29–64

Fig. 29–65

forms either a butt joint or a right angle. It is also advisable to slightly undercut the inner wall of the acrylic periphery with an inverted cone bur.)

21. The inner, or tissue, side of the denture is now sprayed with the first coat of primer (Fig. 29–62), as described under the Multicup procedure, and allowed to bench-dry for 3 minutes.

22. The same area is sprayed a second time and allowed to dry for 3 minutes (Fig. 29–63).

23. Multicup holes are now drilled in the model with a special contra-angle and with a special bur (Fig. 29–64).[1] The model of this denture is now washed with a 10 per-

[1]Suggested by Dr. Arthur C. Jermyn.

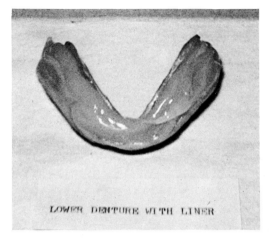

Fig. 29-66

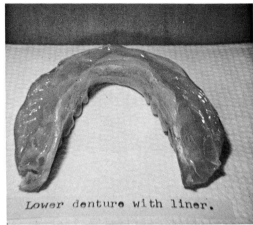

Fig. 29-67

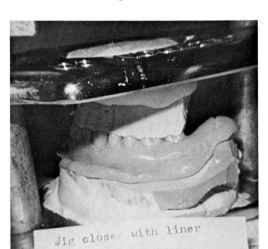

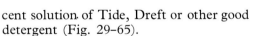

Fig. 29-68

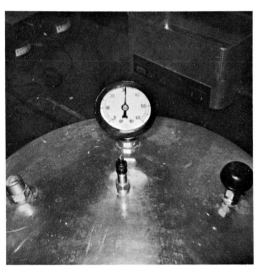

Fig. 29-69

cent solution of Tide, Dreft or other good detergent (Fig. 29-65).

24. At this time prepare the liner material according to the manufacturer's directions and pour it into the primed denture in a way that air pockets are avoided. Slightly overfill (Fig. 29-66).

25. The denture with the soft-filled liner material (Fig. 29-67) is now placed on the model and the jig thoroughly bolted down (Fig. 29-68). The jig is placed in the pres-

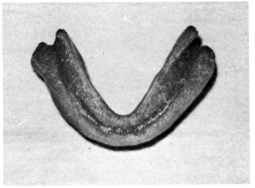

Fig. 29-70

sure cooker in a 165° F water bath, the lid of the cooker is replaced, and 30 lbs. of air pressure is added. It is left to cure at this temperature for 3 hours (Fig. 29–69).

26. After processing, bench-cool for 30 minutes, deflask and trim off the excess flash with a sharp scissors or razor blade.

27. Soak the soft-lined finished denture for 10 minutes (Fig. 29–70) in a mild solution of baking soda to eliminate the slight acetic acid (vinegar) odor.

28. Before dismissing the patient with the new dentures, adjustment of the occlusion is a must. This adjustment is not done in the mouth. Accurate recordings are taken in the mouth and then transferred to an adjustable articulator. Consequently, have the technician make remount models, making certain that the Multicup projections are carefully blocked out with wet tissue paper. Recheck the occlusion with the air-bubble method described in Chapter 23 or, better, use the Baptist apparatus described in Chapters 13 and 33.

29. In order to control bacterial growth on the soft material (Silastic 390), it is advisable to give each patient an ultrasonic denture cleaner kit.[1]

---

[1] Kleen-Dent, Inc.

30

Insertion and Occlusal Adjustment of the Final Processed Dentures Following Tissue Treatment

Because new material was introduced to finalize the tissue-treated dentures, the occlusion must be re-checked under the same conditions as obtained when it was checked originally.

If Porceline was used in the duplication, make use of the remount models made by the technician to repeat the procedure described in Chapter 24. However, if Sofdent was used, the dentures after being processed must soak in water for at least 24 hours in order to soften the Sofdent. While in this soft state, pour the remount models. When these become hard, trim and store them together with the Sofdent-treated dentures in a sealed plastic bag until the patient arrives to

have centric occlusion re-checked. At this point repeat the steps in Chapter 24.

If the Multicup procedure was used, have the patient wear the dentures for a day or two before adjusting the occlusion. At the end of that time, accurate records are taken in the mouth by the use of an intra-oral extra-oral apparatus (Baptist appliance). Using the remount models and face bow record, place the models on an adjustable articulator for occlusal equilibration.

No matter what type of material is used in the final fabrication of the dentures, it is essential to recheck the occlusion by repeating the steps in Chapters 21 through 24.

31
Immediate Dentures

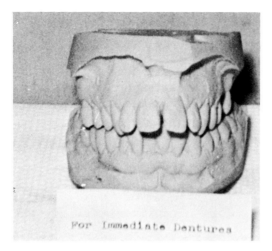

Fig. 31–1

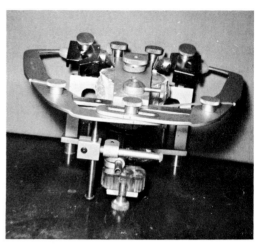

Fig. 31–2

Regardless of what type of dentistry is indicated, it is always advisable to take a full series of X-rays, and a Panorex X-ray. Good study models should be mounted in hinge centric with a face bow record, or, preferably, a pantograph recording should be made and mounted on an arcon instrument (such as the new Denar). Next, a good periodontal examination is made, with pocket depth being fully probed. All factors are evaluated to determine whether complete immediate dentures[1] are necessary. If after a thorough examination, evaluation and patient consultation, we find that they *are* necessary, the following procedure is followed.

(Although it is advisable to make one denture at a time, it is best to make posterior extractions, both maxillary and mandibular, before the replacements.)

1. Extract the upper and lower molars and bicuspids on one side only.

2. Ten days to two weeks later, do the posterior extractions (mandibular and maxillary molars and bicuspids) on the other side. The posterior extractions

[1] I have found it advisable to inform the patient that in order to get best results it is advisable to build immediate dentures first and then make new dentures 9 to 15 months later. (The immediates will then be finalized and kept as spare dentures.)

are done to eliminate an uneven occlusal plane, which may have been caused by a previous drift resulting from the early extraction of teeth that were not replaced.

3. Two or three weeks following the final posterior extractions, take good alginate impressions of the upper and lower jaws (which may retain only the upper and lower anteriors).

4. After pouring these impressions in stone (Fig. 31–1), make upper and lower partial shellac bite blocks.

5. Establish an occlusal plane by using the ala-tragus line, guiding yourself by the incisal edges of the upper incisors.

6. Key the second bicuspid and first molar regions on both sides of the partial upper bite block.

7. Insert this upper bite block in the patient's mouth and, with a bite fork in place, take a face bow record (using the Whip Mix face bow).

8. While the face bow is in place on the

patient's head, observe and record the intercondylar distance on the face bow (S, M or L, as described in Chapter 9).

9. Transfer this face bow record to the Whip Mix articulator (Fig. 31–2).

10. After fitting the upper partial cast into the bite block, articulate this cast to the upper part of the articulator.

11. When the plaster or the stone that was used for securing the cast to the articulator has set, remove the face bow apparatus from the instrument and separate the face bow from the upper bite block.

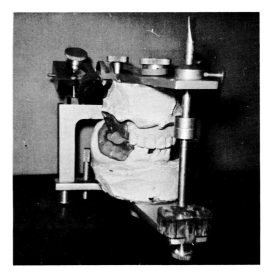

Fig. 31–3

12. Remembering to place petrolatum on the key areas, replace this upper keyed bite block in the patient's mouth.

13. Adjust the lower partial bite block by trimming down the wax. This is done to the extent that when they are placed in the patient's mouth, and he is asked to close upon both upper and lower bite blocks, the upper and lower jaws almost come together, and the upper and lower anterior teeth meet in normal occlusion.

14. Trim down the wax on the lower bite block about 3 mm. more. This leaves a space between the upper and lower bite blocks in the posterior region.

15. Place a small mound of wax 6 to 8 mm. in height on both sides of the lower bite block opposite the keys of the upper bite block.

16. Drape a piece of the same wax (Wafer Wax, Modern Materials), about 4 mm. in height and 6 mm. in length, over the incisal edges of the patient's lower anterior incisors.

17. With a torch, slightly heat the mounds of wax on the lower bite block.

18. Insert the lower bite block in the mouth.

19. Place a wafer candy in the patient's mouth and permit him to swallow into centric occlusion.

Note: At this point I must urge you to eliminate muscle spasm, as was done in Chapter 9. Also, because the anterior teeth may act as guiding influences, check swallowing procedure; chill and remove the bite blocks and the anterior wax "drape" just before the patient brings the lingual surfaces of the anterior teeth into contact.

20. Transfer these records to the articulator, which retains the previously articulated upper model.

21. Finish the articulation (Fig. 31–3).

22. Select the shade and mold (Fig. 31–4).

23. Set up the upper posterior teeth (Fig. 31–5).

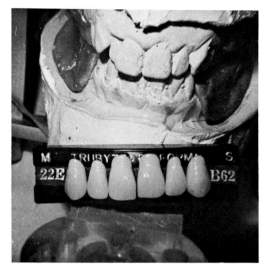

Fig. 31–4

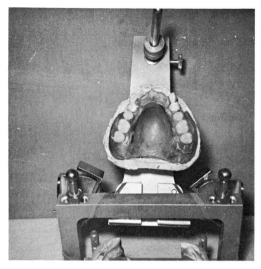

Fig. 31–5

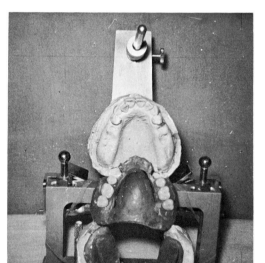

Fig. 31–6

26. When adding the denture teeth to the bite block, cut out every other tooth on the stone cast until you have completed the anterior set-up. Any modifications in esthetics are readily made at this time. When the upper immediate wax set-up is completed (Fig. 31–8) it is best to make a face bow record (Fig. 31–9), which will be used when you make the lower immediate denture and also when rechecking centric later on.

27. Remove the upper model and wax denture from the articulator and send it to the laboratory with instructions to finish the upper denture by butting the anterior teeth (with no labial flange) (Fig. 31–10). Also, instruct the technician to take an alginate impression of the occlusal surfaces of the finished upper denture.

24. Try in this upper partial wax try-in to check the line-up of the occlusal plane (Fig. 31–6).

25. If everything checks out—and it should—add the anterior teeth to this partial bite block by first cutting off one of the stone centrals from the cast and replacing it with a denture tooth (Fig. 31–7).

28. A stone model is made of this alginate impression. This will be used during the making of the lower immediate denture.

29. After the technician has returned the finished upper case, call in the patient. Using a local anesthetic, extract (or have the oral surgeon extract) the remaining anterior teeth.

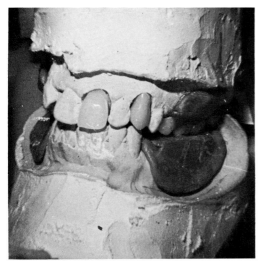

Fig. 31-7

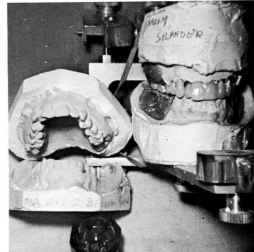

Fig. 31-8

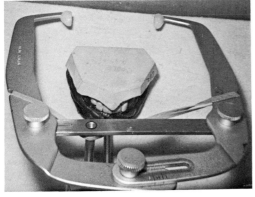

Fig. 31-9

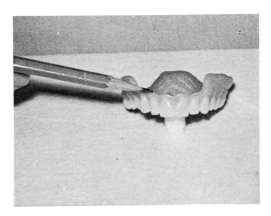

Fig. 31-10

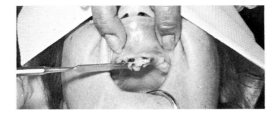

Fig. 31-11

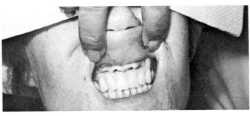

Fig. 31-12

30. Immediately following these extractions I place an antibiotic in each socket [such as Terramycin Dental Cones (Pfizer)] covered with either Kenalog in Orabase (Squibb) or Cortisporin (Burroughs Wellcome) (Fig. 31-11). By means of this drug therapy, I have for many years been able to control edema and increase patient comfort.

31. Try-in the upper finished denture (Fig. 31-12). If the technician used a careful processing procedure this denture

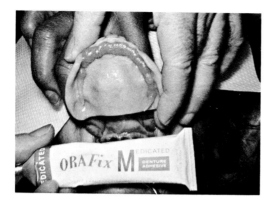

Fig. 31-13

should fit well. In most cases no adjustments should be necessary. However, if some are, they should be minor.

32. When satisfied with the fit, remove the denture from the mouth and place Ora-Fix[1] (Fig. 31-13).

33. Instruct the patient to eat soft foods and not to remove the denture. He should return to the office the following day for a check-up.

34. When he does, remove the denture and instruct him on thorough brushing.

35. Have him insert a generous amount of the Ora-Fix medication himself and replace the denture in the mouth himself.

36. Instruct him to remove and brush the denture and to replace the medication each morning and night. Also tell him to keep the denture in his mouth 24 hours a day, removing it only for brushing and the replacement of the medication. Have him return to the office one week later.

37. At this next visit, remove the medication and paint tissue treatment (Hydro-Cast, or a similar material) on the inside of the denture.

[1] Norcliff Labs., Fairfield, Conn.

38. Tell him *not* to brush this upper denture, but to remove it twice a day and rinse it off under cold tap water. He should return to the office one week later. (This visit will be for a change of treatment and for work on the lower immediate denture.)

39. When he returns to the office, pour a model of the upper tissue-treated denture and occlusal index. Place in the jig in order to perform the procedure as done in Chapter 27.

40. Remove the denture from the jig, make a new mix of tissue treatment, and paint it over the entire area. Insert the denture in the mouth as done in Chapter 27 (Step 20).

41. After 8 minutes, remove from the mouth and trim off the excess.

42. Now take the lower previously prepared bite block and place mounds of soft wax (Modern Materials) about 4 mm. in height in the molar and bicuspid regions on both sides.

43. Place a mound of this same wax about 5 mm. in height on the centrals of the upper denture.

44. After slightly heating the mounds of wax on the lower bite block, insert into the patient's mouth and register centric (as was done in Step 19). Once again you must make sure the patient is free of muscle spasms.

45. When centric relation has been recorded, chill and remove.

46. Use the original face bow transfer (or take a new face bow transfer using the upper denture) and, after taking an

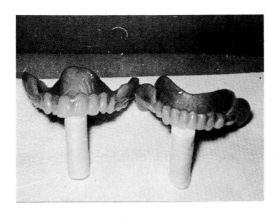

Fig. 31–14

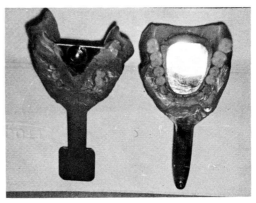

Fig. 31–15

alginate impression of the occlusal surface of the upper denture, pour a model and insert this model into the face bow record.

47. Articulate the lower partial bite block to this upper model.

48. Set up the lower posterior teeth to the upper model.

49. Try-in the lower posterior set-up in the patient's mouth.

50. Finish the lower anterior set-up by repeating Steps 25 and 26 (done for the upper anteriors).

51. Remove the lower wax denture on the model from the articulator and send it to the laboratory with instructions to finish by butting the anterior teeth (with no labial flange) (Fig. 31–14).

52. Repeat Steps 29 through 39.

53. New stone models may now be poured into these tissue treated dentures and the tissue treatments changed.

54. Remove both dentures from the jigs and proceed as in Chapter 27.

55. Make a new mix (one part liquid to one part powder).

56. Immediately paint this mixture completely over the tissue-treated surfaces of both dentures, like a wash over a wash.

57. Reinsert both dentures in the patient's mouth and have him hold in occlusion for 3 minutes.

58. At the end of about 8 minutes, remove both dentures from the patient's mouth and trim off the excess tissue treatment.

59. Reinsert the dentures and dismiss the patient with instructions to return one week later for a change of treatment and equilibration of the occlusion.

60. When the patient returns, remove the tissue-treated dentures from the mouth (Fig. 31–14) and insert the intra-oral extra-oral apparatus (as was done in the case of anterior teeth only in Chapter 13) (Fig. 31–15). This time we are going to repeat that procedure but on a complete full upper and lower.

61. Record centric occlusion position and then the eccentric positions of the right and left laterals. Before introducing the fast

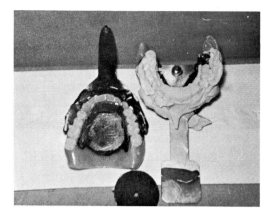

Fig. 31–16

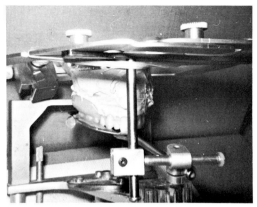

Fig. 31–17

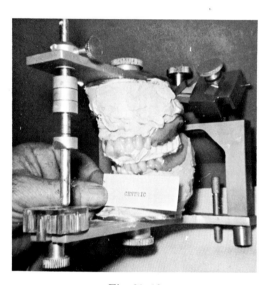

Fig. 31–18

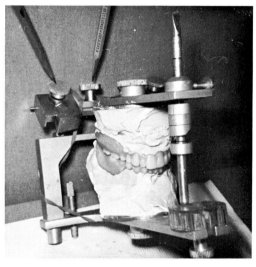

Fig. 31–19

setting stone for these positions, the soft rubber sponge of the Baptist apparatus is inserted between the upper and lower apparatuses in order to equalize the pressure on the ridges (Fig. 31–16).

62. After taking the check bites, dismantle the apparatus and pour new stone models into these tissue-treated cases.

63. By first using the previous face bow record, or by taking a new record (Fig. 31–17), mount the case on the Whip Mix articulator with a centric check bite (Fig. 31–18).

64. Now by using the lateral stone check bite wafers, individually, set the articulator for the right and then the left lateral movements. These check bites, automatically, have recorded, to some degree, the Bennett movements and condylar inclinations (Fig. 31–19).

65. While they are on the articulator, adjust the dentures to a balanced occlusion as was done in Chapter 24.

66. After the dentures have been balanced, remove each model with the denture on it.

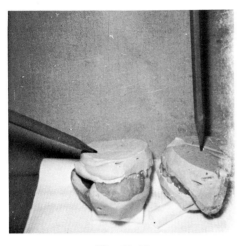

Fig. 31–20

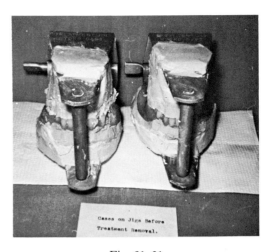

Fig. 31–21

67. Make a new index model of the incisal and occlusal surfaces of each denture (Fig. 31–20).

68. Articulate each denture into a separate jig (Fig. 31–21).

69. When the plaster on the articulated jig has set, open the jig and remove each denture from its seat (Fig. 31–22).

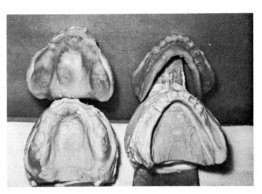

Fig. 31–22

70. After removing the old tissue treatment material from each denture with a No. 12 round bur, and scrapers, continue with the same procedure used in Chapter 27 (Steps 9 through 20). However, in the case of immediate dentures, it is necessary to see the patient about once a month for a change of tissue treatment. During this period of therapy, use the same jigs, and each time the tissue treatment is removed from these dentures repeat Steps 9 through 20 in Chapter 27.

71. Nine to 15 months following the extractions and the tissue treatment, these dentures may be made permanent, or new dentures made and these treatment dentures kept as spares. I advise my patients to have new dentures made at the end of the 9 to 15 month period.

32

The Full Upper Denture Against the Lower Natural or Partial Dentition

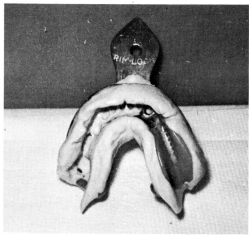

Fig. 32–1

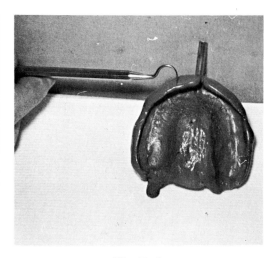

Fig. 32–2

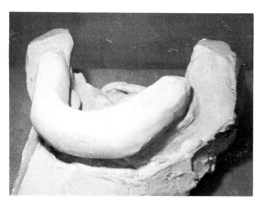

Fig. 32–3

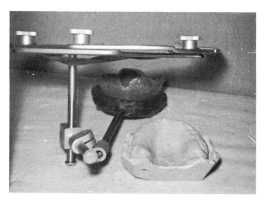

Fig. 32–4

In building a full upper denture against the patient's own natural or partial lower dentition, the same procedure is followed, with some minor alterations or additions, as in the building of full upper and lower dentures.

After a thorough evaluation of the case —including X-rays, study models, checking for muscle spasms, and a periodontal examination of the remaining teeth—we are ready to build the full upper denture.

1. Take a good preliminary alginate impression of the maxillary edentulous ridge as well as one of the lower full dentition. If the patient is wearing a good fitting lower partial appliance, take the impression with that appliance in place (Fig. 32–1).

2. Obtain an upper wash impression by following the steps in Chapter 4, using either the EX-3-N or a rubber base material (Fig. 32–2).

3. At this time make an acrylic onlay type of apparatus (Fig. 32–3) from the lower cast impression and store for future use in recording centric and eccentric positions (which is not necessary if a new lower partial is to be constructed).

4. After the upper bite block is made from this wash impression, begin the next phase by following Steps 1 to 10 in Chapter 9. Also refer to Chapter 10 and 11 for the shaping of the upper anterior bite block and the selection of the anterior teeth.

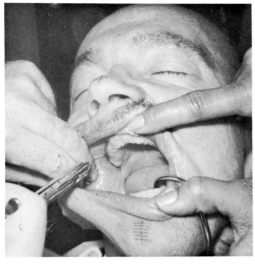

Fig. 32-5

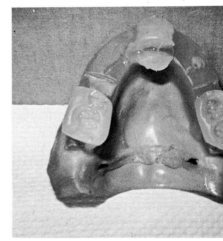

Fig. 32-6

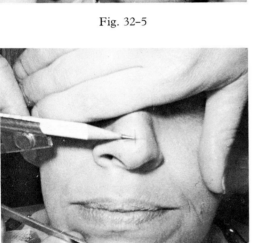

Fig. 32-7

Fig. 32-8

5. Once the rest position and the correct amount of freeway space have been established, cut down the height of the wax of this bite block to make allowance for these measurements.

6. Now follow the complete outline of steps in Chapters 7 and 8. Take a face bow record of upper (Fig. 32-4) and articulate to the upper part of Whip Mix articulator.

7. You are now ready to record vertical and tentative centric occlusion by the act of swallowing. Again you must check for muscle spasms (Fig. 32-5). However, at this time, cut down the upper posterior section of the bite block about 2 to 3 mm. from first biscuspid back towards the tuberosity. After placing the wafer wax in the three areas, the molar and anterior regions, and with a candy in the mouth (Fig. 32-6), allow the patient to swallow in upon this soft wax.

8. After the patient has swallowed into vertical and tentative centric relation (Fig. 32-7), remove the swallowed-in up-

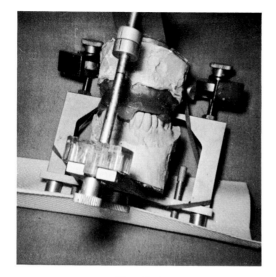

Fig. 32–9

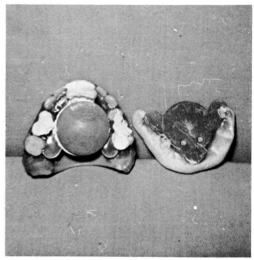

Fig. 32–10

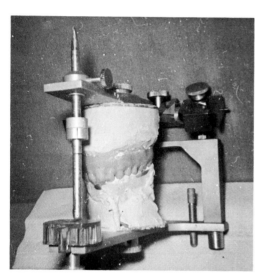

Fig. 32–11

Fig. 32–12

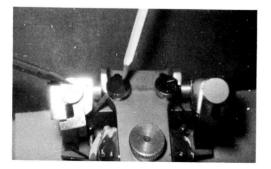

Fig. 32–13

per (Fig. 32–8) from the mouth and finish the articulation (Fig. 32–9).

9. Set up the 6 anterior teeth (Fig. 32–10) using the same principles as in Chapter 11.

10. Try-in this 6 upper anterior set up in the mouth and check esthetics and phonetics (Chapter 12).

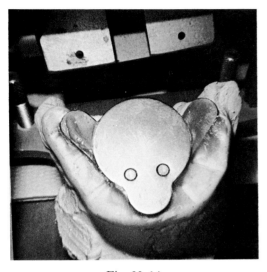

Fig. 32-14

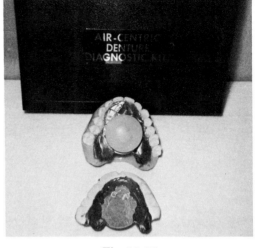

Fig. 32-15

11. Follow the steps in Chapter 13.

12. Follow the steps in Chapter 14.

13. Follow the steps in Chapter 15.

14. Finish setting the upper posterior teeth against the lower (Fig. 32-11).

15. Follow the steps in Chapter 17. (Fig. 32-12).

16. Balance the case by following the steps in Chapter 18 (Fig. 32-13).

17. Follow the steps in Chapters 21, 22 and 23. When the upper case has been returned by the laboratory, the technician should be instructed to make a remount model for this upper denture.

18. Attaching the lower platform to the lower acrylic overlay (Fig. 32-14), and attaching the diagnostic air bubble to the palate of the upper (Fig. 32-15), recheck centric occlusion in the mouth, as was done in Chapter 24.

19. Follow the steps in Chapter 24. The one variation is that Temp-Bond is on the upper denture.

20. Follow the steps in Chapters 26 and 27.

21. Follow the steps under "A" in Chapter 29.

22. Follow the steps in Chapter 30.

33

Salvaging Full Upper and Lower Dentures That Are Troublesome

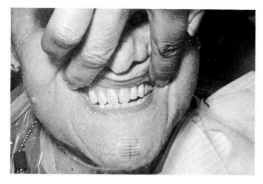

Fig. 33–1

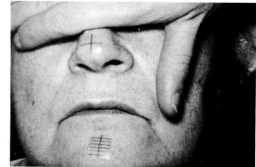

Fig. 33–2

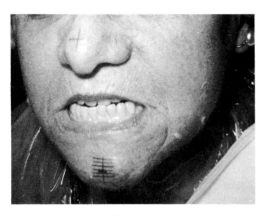

Fig. 33–3

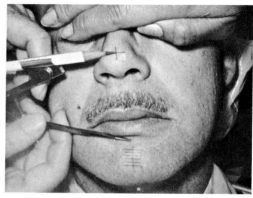

Fig. 33–4

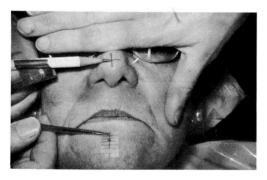

Fig. 33–5

Some of us have had the unpleasant experience of building full upper and lower dentures that appeared to be satisfactory because the patient was willing, for the first two or three months, to accustom himself to the dentures that were not comfortable.

Upon checking the centric position, we find that this patient's dentures are not only out of centric occlusion, but have assumed a pseudo Class III malocclusion, or protrusive position (Fig. 33–1). Why? What caused this position to be assumed? At this point you must evaluate all factors that may be responsible for the patient's discomfort, and determine whether rebuilding the lower denture only might salvage the case to some satisfactory level. To do this, the following procedure is undertaken.

1. Place a piece of tape with a "+" mark on the nose, and another piece on the chin bearing one vertical line intersected by 5 or 6 horizontal lines about 2 mm. apart (Fig. 33–2).

2. Ask the patient to close and hold with the teeth in contact in the acquired Class III position (Fig. 33–3).

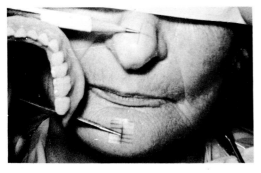

Fig. 33–6

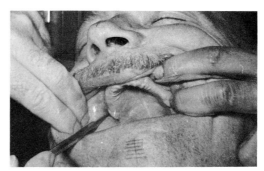

Fig. 33–7

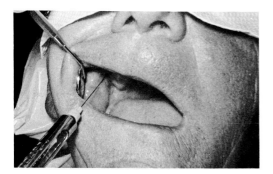

Fig. 33–8

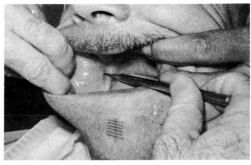

Fig. 33–9

3. With a pair of calipers, measure the distance between the "+" mark on the nose and the uppermost horizontal line on the chin (Fig. 33–4).

4. Remove the lower denture from his mouth and measure the rest position. Note the measurement when both dentures are in the mouth (Fig. 33–5) vs. the measurement when the lower denture is out of the mouth. In most cases we find that the freeway space has been encroached upon (Fig. 33–6).

5. Palpate the attachments of the right and left external pterygoid fibers (Fig. 33–7). These muscles will be in spasm as a rule, and this should be eliminated (Fig. 33–8).

6. Palpate the attachments of the internal pterygoid fibers (Fig. 33–9) and relieve any spasm (Fig. 33–10).

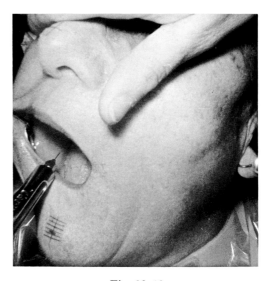

Fig. 33–10

7. Wait 5 to 10 minutes before rechecking the dentures in the mouth. Observe how the patient goes back into centric occlusion and interdigitates the dentures (Fig.

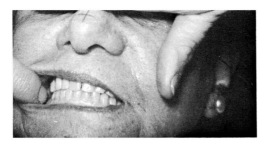

Fig. 33-11

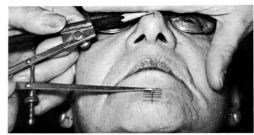

Fig. 33-12

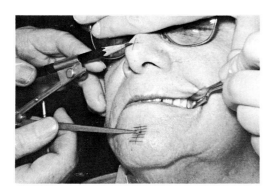

Fig. 33-13

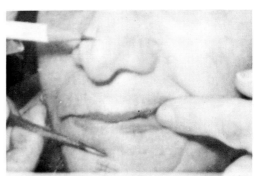

Fig. 33-14

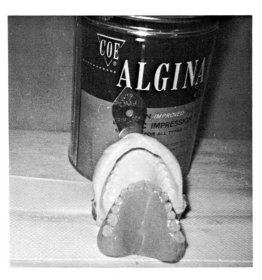

Fig. 33-15

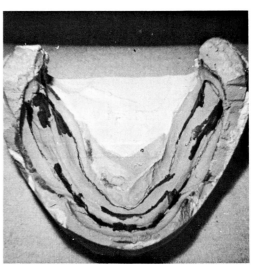

Fig. 33-16

33-11). Recheck the rest position (Fig. 33-12) with the calipers.

8. Recheck freeway space (Fig. 33-13) and compare it to the dimensional open-

ing present in your original case (Fig. 33-14). By releasing the muscle spasms the jaw has been permitted to give us the correct freeway space.

We now find that in most of these pseudo Class III cases, not only was the

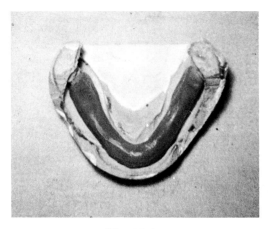

Fig. 33-17

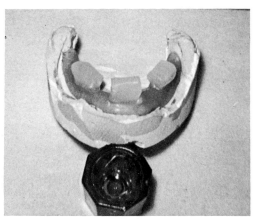

Fig. 33-18

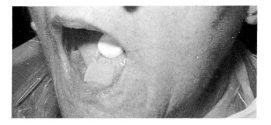

Fig. 33-19

freeway space not provided for, but we actually jeopardized the rest position. When we have the jaws in terminal hinge position, there is a certain height of opening between the jaws. However, as the patient moves his jaws into a protrusive position, the amount of jaw separation is reduced. Because we permitted too much jaw separation, the muscular apparatus became tired and tried to relieve the strain by pushing the lower jaw out protrusively, thereby slightly closing the dimension. However, when the jaw does this, an occlusal problem is introduced by the movement of the dentures. If the patient puts up with this condition for any length of time, the bone structures supporting the soft tissues begin to resorb. Eventually we have very little foundation upon which to build a satisfactory denture.

Therefore, if we have made these dentures within the last 6 to 12 months, we can attempt to salvage them by redoing only the lower. A special "shortcut" method can be used, tissue-treating both upper and lower dentures at the same time, and finalizing both dentures, using Porceline as the rebase.

1. Take an alginate impression (Fig. 33-15) of the patient's upper denture and pour this impression in stone.

2. Take a good preliminary alginate impression of the patient's lower ridge.

3. After blocking out some of the bad undercuts with soft wax or Plastercine (Fig. 33-16), construct a pink acrylic tray.

4. Place two sheets of a hard wax (Fig. 33-17) on this acrylic tray, making an acrylic bite block.

5. Place three mounds of soft wafer wax (Fig. 33-18) on the molars and on the anterior regions of this low acrylic bite block.

6. Replace the upper denture in the mouth, the incisal and occlusal surfaces covered with petrolatum.

7. Slightly heat the three wax areas on the lower bite block with an alcohol torch. Insert in the patient's mouth.

8. Place wafer candy on the patient's tongue (Fig. 33-19) with instructions to swallow the saliva whenever he feels it necessary to do so.

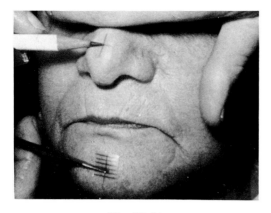

Fig. 33–20

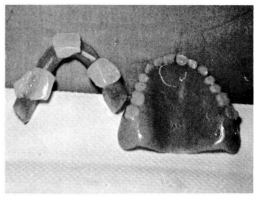

Fig. 33–21

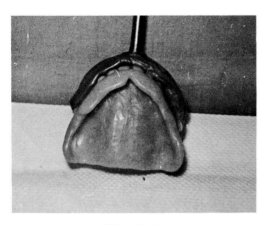

Fig. 33–22

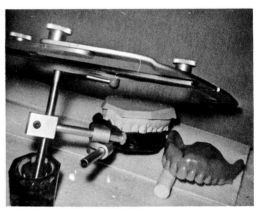

Fig. 33–23

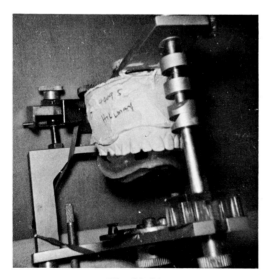

Fig. 33–24

9. At the end of 5 or 10 minutes, because the patient's internal and external pterygoids spasm regions have been eliminated, he will swallow into the correct vertical (Fig. 33–20) and tentative centric relation.

10. Chill the wax with ice water, separate the bite block from the upper denture (Fig. 33–21) and remove both from mouth.

11. Take a face bow mounting (Fig. 33–22) of the upper denture in the mouth.

12. Place the stone cast originally taken of the upper denture into the face bow

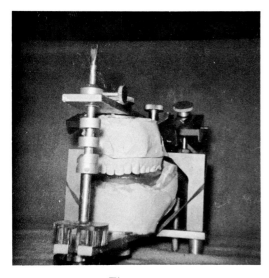

Fig. 33-25

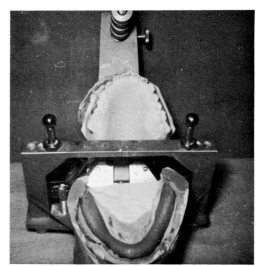

Fig. 33-26

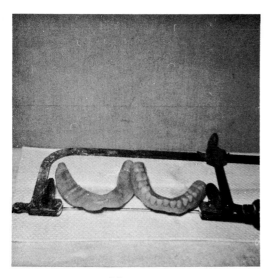

Fig. 33-27

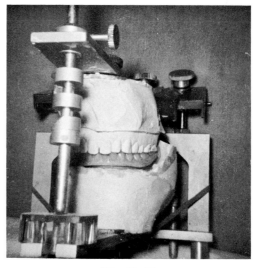

Fig. 33-28

record (Fig. 33-23) and articulate this to the upper part of the articulator.

13. Position the low wax indented acrylic bite block in relation to this upper and, fitting the lower cast (Fig. 33-24) to the acrylic bite block, finish the articulation (Fig. 33-25).

14. When the plaster has set, remove the three stops of soft wafer wax from the acrylic bite block (Fig. 33-26).

15. With a saw, cut off the teeth of the lower denture in a block (Fig. 33-27) and fit them on the acrylic block (Fig. 33-28) of the lower, first removing all wax adhering to the acrylic tray. It may be necessary to grind away a great deal of the old acrylic from this block in order to fit it over the area and into interdigitation against the upper stone model.

16. When properly in place, tag this block

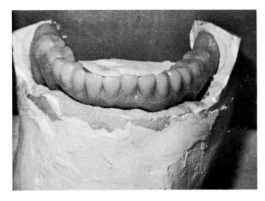

Fig. 33–29

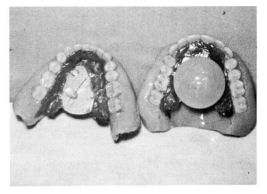

Fig. 33–30

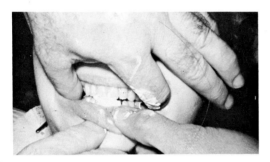

Fig. 33–31

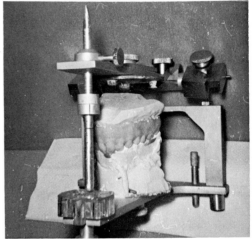

Fig. 33–32

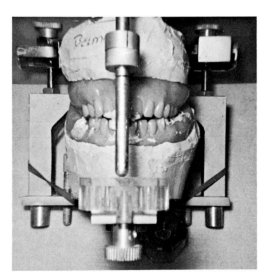

Fig. 33–33

lower (Fig. 33–29) and place the air bubble apparatus between the palate of the patient's upper denture and the platform of the apparatus in the lower denture (Fig. 33–30) preparatory to taking an equalization record in the mouth.

18. Using Temp-Bond, and with the jaw in hinge centric position, take a centric record only (Fig. 33–31).

19. Articulate this position by using the original indexed face bow record to mount the upper denture with the remount model (Fig. 33–32), and remount the lower denture with the Temp-Bond record (Fig. 33–33).

of teeth to the new acrylic base by means of fast-set powder and liquid acrylic.

17. When the acrylic has set, polish the

20. Equilibrate the occlusion in centric position only. At this point, those who wish to achieve an even greater degree of refinement in occlusal function may take eccentric check bites by using the principles described in Chapter 13.

21. After the occlusal adjustments have been completed on the articulator, prepare the case to receive the first tissue treatment material, as described in Chapter 27. It should not be necessary to treat this type of case over any more than four visits.

22. At the end of the tissue treatment procedure, duplicate the upper and lower by using the Porceline procedure described in Chapter 30.

23. Recheck the occlusion at insertion time, following the procedure described in Chapter 31.

34

Gnathologic Principles in Complete Denture Construction

by Peter K. Thomas, D.D.S.
Leo McCallum, D.D.S.
Robert J. Pinkerton, D.D.S.
Roy Taylor, D.D.S. and
Jack M. Buchman, D.D.S.

THE MEANING OF GNATHOLOGY

Gnathology is a relatively new term, recently derived, which appears to mean different things to different practitioners; even "gnathologists" differ among themselves. As originally defined by Beverly B. McCollum, the term means "the science that treats of the biologies of the masticatory mechanism, that is, the morphology, anatomy, histology, physiology, pathology, and therapeutics of the oral organ, especially the jaws and teeth and the vital relations of this organ to the rest of the body."[1] In essence, this is really a definition of Dentistry and does not describe the specifics of gnathology as it is practiced today.

Another interesting definition of gnathology is that of Dr. Niles F. Guichet of California. "Gnathology has as its foundation a rationale of diagnosis and treatment of the gnatho-stomatic system based on a comprehensive understanding of the etiologic nature of stress as it relates to dental disease. It has to do with the treatment of the oral cavity and related structures as an integrated organ rather than as a collection of unrelated components."[2] Here again, we have a definition that skirts the frequent rejection of some very useful principles because these principles are prefaced by the term gnathology.

In truth, gnathology as practiced today is a meticulous, mechanistic study of temporomandibular movements, selective measuring of such movements, and, finally, graphically reproducing them so that they may be used in the diagnosis and treatment of occlusion. Gnathology is essentially a search for precision in the recording and fabrication of an optimum occlusion for the individual patient. There is no question in our minds that it has earned a place in the armamentarium of the careful practitioner who is interested in objective procedures that offer greater accuracy in the analysis and treatment of occlusion, and that hopefully make the outcome more predictable.

[1] McCollum, B. B.: Fundamentals involved in prescribing restorative dental remedies. Dental Items of Interest, *61*:522, 1939.
[2] Guichet, Niles F.: Gnathology—Everyday Dentistry. 1966.

PRINCIPLES OF GNATHOLOGY

Gnathology has its greatest effect and use in restorative dentistry because jaw movements are what they are, whether you are treating the natural dentition, performing complete rehabilitation, or inserting complete dentures. Whatever resides in that mouth is going to be treated kindly, or is going to be badly abused, depending upon its relationship to the prevailing jaw movements and the harmony, or lack of harmony, therein.

Although in the past some of the far-reaching effects of occlusal stress have gone largely unrecognized or unappreciated, we know that deflective cuspal inclines in natural teeth have been identified as a source of tooth mobility, and deflective cuspal inclines in complete dentures have been recognized as dislodging factors of the denture base. Aside from the dislodging factors involved in deflective denture cusp inclines, there is also the possibility that the patient will attempt to accommodate to his denture malocclusion by assuming an adjusted postural position of the mandible. This is an attempt by the fourth determinant of mandibular movement—the patient's neuromusculature—to cause the teeth to come into a more even or harmonious relationship. Generally it is accomplished through a downward–forward–lateral repositioning of the mandible. The net effect of this adjusted postural position is a lessening of the fulcruming forces applied to the interfering inclines.

If this were all that occurred within the gnathostomatic system during the accommodation, it could be agreed that the accommodation has served a useful biologic function. However, it is necessary for one or the other of the external pterygoid muscles and associated muscle groups to be under a heavy perpetual state of contraction to effect the postural repositioning. This leads to a considerable amount of discomfort, pain and inability to function normally as the muscles enter a condition of spasm. The postural accommodation effected by one group of muscles can have an overriding effect upon other groups of muscles in the head and neck region, thus giving rise to muscular soreness and aches in these regions. It is entirely possible that certain head, neck and upper shoulder pain is related to an underlying occlusal dysfunction. Certainly in complete denture construction there are many mechanical limitations imposed upon the operator that are beyond his control.

In order to have denture base stability during functional movement it is generally considered necessary to provide some form of a balanced scheme of occlusion. The following should be incorporated into the optimal occlusion for complete denture construction:

1. The criteria of good centric occlusion.

2. Adequate lateral contact in eccentric positions to provide stability.

3. Adequate steepness of posterior cusps to reduce vertical overloading.

4. Provision for a tolerance in the occlusion in the lateral dimensions so that mandibular movement in that direction does not cause premature cusp contact.

A denture occlusion fabricated in accord with these criteria exert the minimal amount of stress on the underlying ridges, musculature and temporomandibular joints during functional movements of the mandible.

Clinical Application of Gnathologic Principles—Instrumentation, Interpretation and Procedures

Our chief concern in denture contruction is to provide our patients with aesthetically acceptable, comfortable, correctly functioning dentures, so designed as to protect and preserve the underlying tissues as long as physiologically possible. To accomplish this there are myriad tasks that must be effectively accomplished. Foremost among these is the effective capture, transfer and use of the individual, anatomically correct, maxillomandibular relation for this patient, most usually designated as "centric relation." Gnathologically speaking, the term centric relation is synonymous with the terminal hinge position, further defined as the most retruded relation of the mandible to the maxilla when the condyles are rearmost, uppermost, and midmost in the glenoid fossa. The hinge axis is found within the terminal hinge position and it is a retruded, vertical, nonfunctional arcing that is consistently repeatable.

We must have a starting base from which we proceed to measure or custom-fit our patient, a reference point to which we can return with assurance. We cannot set up teeth, process them and recheck them in the patient's mouth. We must use a laboratory instrument, an articulator, to help us. Theoretically, the closer this instrument comes to duplicating the physiology and anatomy of the patient, the more confidence we can have that what we construct on it will be suitable for the patient. For example, the dentist who satisfactorily registers the fine detail of his crown preparation fully expects the returned finished product to fit the tooth for which it was constructed, if the steps subsequent to impression-taking were carefully followed. He knows that by so doing a duplicate of the patient's tooth has been captured, thus providing himself or his technician with a convenient vehicle upon which to construct whatever is required. The objective, then, in a set of dentures, is to faithfully capture that relation of the mandible to the maxilla in the correct position essential to fabricate an occlusion that will meet the criteria we have already established.

But that is only step number one. The test comes in transferring the specific relations from our patient to our instrument, first with fidelity and then with high confidence that the instrument can accept the information we put into it and can return to us precisely this same information in a mechanically usable fashion to satisfy the physiologic needs of the patient.

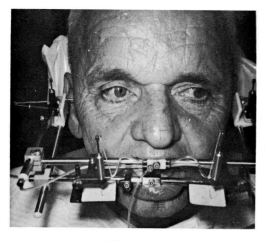

Fig. 34–1

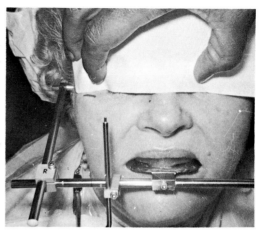

Fig. 34–2

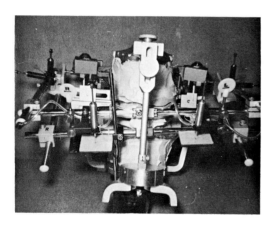

Fig. 34–3

It is our belief that for the utmost in denture construction, gnathology offers some of the best instrumentation available.

Gnathological instruments are essentially three in number:

1. A pantograph (Fig. 34–1).

2. An adjustable face bow and hinge axis recorder (Fig.34–2).

3. A fully adjustable articulator (Fig. 34–3).

The gnathologic purist considers all of these instruments necessary. There are many, however, who use gnathologic principles without employing the full range of specialized instruments and, with only a few exceptions, achieve optimum results in full denture construction.

The Pantograph

A pantograph is an instrument for the mechanical copying to scale of plan, motion, and function. In our field, the pantograph copies or reproduces the effects of the axes of rotations and translations of the mandible in border positions. These effects are written on horizontal and vertical plates located in the region of the temporomandibular joint and in the anterolateral segment region of the mandible. The quickest and most easily applicable pantograph in our experience is the Denar pantograph.[1]

Since the condyles travel along multiple paths, and since a free-functioning mandible travels an infinite number of paths within its range of movement, one might feel that a fully functional recorder and articulator would be ideal. But how could any instrument handle an infinite number of movements? Thus, in the absence of such instrumentation, the utilization of an existing writing instrument, the pantograph, becomes our concern.

Remember that the pantograph copies

[1]Denar Corp., 2220 Howell St., Anaheim, Cal.

what exists, which may not be correct function. Should the patient's temporomandibular joints and associated structures be in spasm, the areas must first be detected and treated before recordings are taken. It is the dentist's responsibility to evaluate the patient's physiology before having the instrument record.

If we assume that the patient has a correctly functioning neuromuscular system, the pantograph is currently the most accurate method available to us for recording the anatomic characteristics of the temporomandibular articulations having an influence on the projected occlusion.

Built into almost every procedure we know today are certain inaccuracies—system errors, so to speak. Utilization of a pantograph requires rigid fixation of the clutches to the upper and lower jaws for accurate reproductions. Thus, in complete dentures, where we are dealing with movable, unstable, edentulous areas, difficulty in stabilizing the pantograph is a potential source of system error we cannot ignore. The accuracy of our recordings depends on whether we are working with high, well-formed ridges with tightly attached mucosal tissues or low, poorly formed, flabby ridges (remembering of course, that these factors exert their influence no matter what method we employ to gather our necessary jaw relation records). The pantograph serves us best when it diagnoses for us the essential character of lateral movement, its very path and sometimes unique curvature. It serves us well and is often worth the effort and time needed to utilize it when, for example, it graphically highlights for us an immediate side shift in the rotating condyle, in lateral movement—the so-called Bennett movement. It is this movement, or, we might better say, the character of this movement, that is a frequent source of difficulty to both the patient and dentist in reconstructive procedures, whether it be in the dentulous or edentulous mouth.

If the patient has an immediate bodily shift of the mandible at the beginning of the lateral stroke, it is essential that the cusps which form the occlusal contacting surfaces of the dentition have a small area in which they can move without contacting one another. If this movement is not provided for in the restored occlusion, there will be constant interference on the balancing side and the patient will experience consistent soreness beneath the interfering teeth, resorption of the ridges and excessive tooth wear, in the case of acrylic teeth, or frequent breakage or chipping, in the case of porcelain teeth.

Fortunately, marked immediate side-shifts are not common findings. The check-bite technique cannot capture this phenomenon. A check-bite record, no matter what the recording medium, is a positional registration; it will tell you the character of mandibular movement only at the position recorded. The check-bite, or pin, method results in a straight horizontal guide on the articulator. By comparison, the pantograph precisely records the character of the emenentia and results in a customized guide on the articulator.

The Adjustable Face Bow and Hinge Axis Recorder

In preparing the case for our work the upper cast must be correctly oriented to the opening axis of the articulator just as the maxilla is to the skull. To accomplish the transferring of this relationship, we employ the face bow. The true hinge axis is located by use of an adjustable caliper-like instrument that may be part of, or supplement to, the face bow. Location is accomplished by a series of controlled opening and closing movements of the mandible when it is in the terminal hinge position. This location is the first step in the correct transfer of centric relation from the patient to the instrument. Theoretically, and to some extent on a practical basis, we can locate the true hinge axis. But we must not get "hung up" on this procedure. Sometimes, the pinpoint accuracy demanded by advocates of pure gnathologic concepts makes a fetish of this point; however there are limitations to our ability to capture this very small area. It demands not only the coordinated efforts of both the patient and the dentist, but also a completely relaxed patient and a completely relaxed dentist, and a healthy, properly functioning neuromusculature.

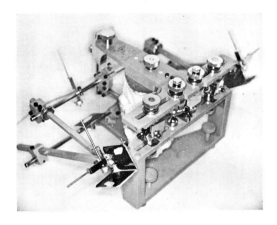

Fig. 34–4

Location of the true hinge axis is required if we wish to change the vertical dimension between the casts on the articulator and still maintain the same centric relation without going back to the mouth. It is also required if the casts are transferred to the articulator at an increased vertical dimension. If, however, the centric relation record is obtained at the correct vertical dimension, a selected hinge axis registration is sufficient and can eliminate many of the errors associated with location and transfer of the true hinge axis. For this reason a less sophisticated but very practical articulator, the Whip Mix articulator, finds a definite place in the resources of the dentist interested in gnathologic principles but not necessarily in complete gnathological instrumentation. This instrument is capable of accepting a true hinge axis recording and provides a rapid method for locating and transferring a selected axis by the use of a quick-mount face bow. It is an arcon instrument and can be set quickly and satisfactorily in most instances by use of check-bite recordings. While it will not satisfactorily accept a pantograph, this is, in principle, a utilization of gnathologic concepts. Hinge axis recordings are taken, an arcon instrument

is used, and cognizance is taken of the lateral movements, with some possibility of allowing for Bennett movement.

The Articulator

This is a controversial subject, and the question of "which articulator" still debated. Our discussion here is related to gnathologic concepts, and in such a discussion the choice of articulator plays a vital role. It would avail us little to secure a pantographic tracing to place on an instrument incapable of either receiving it or reproducing the movements recorded.

An articulator is a mechanical device by which movements of the temporomandibular joints and mandible can be simulated to obtain proper relationships of teeth in occlusion. It should have capabilities of receiving and registering those crania-to-jaw and jaw-to-jaw relations. More important, not only should it receive such recordings, it should allow the operator the freedom to program its controls in such a way as to insure the fabrication of the desired occlusion.

There are at present several fully adjustable instruments, of which the Stuart instrument (Fig. 34–4) is the most accurate, capable of producing all the details of a pantographic tracing.[1]

For ease of manipulation, many of us favor the use of the new Denar D4A articulator for the more complicated cases, with the use of the true hinge recordings, although an arbitary axis may sometimes be employed. This articulator can also be used as a check-bite instrument. Several other instruments are capable of accepting the pantograph, but we question their ability to completely follow the tracings.

---

[1] The Stuart Cusp Computer, the Ney Articulator, the Granger Gnatholator, and the Denar D4A Articulator.

35

Construction of Full Upper and Lower Dentures Employing the Denar Pantograph and the Denar D4A Articulator

By Robert J. Pinkerton, D.D.S. and
Jack M. Buchman, D.D.S.

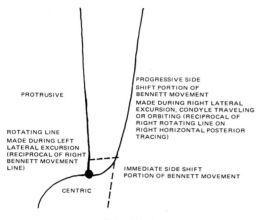

PROTRUSIVE

PROGRESSIVE SIDE
SHIFT PORTION OF
BENNETT MOVEMENT
MADE DURING RIGHT LATERAL
EXCURSION, CONDYLE TRAVELING
OR ORBITING (RECIPROCAL OF
RIGHT ROTATING LINE ON
RIGHT HORIZONTAL POSTERIOR
TRACING)

ROTATING LINE
MADE DURING LEFT
LATERAL EXCURSION
(RECIPROCAL OF RIGHT
BENNETT MOVEMENT
LINE)

IMMEDIATE SIDE SHIFT
PORTION OF BENNETT MOVEMENT

CENTRIC

Fig. 35–1

Since I am now a strong believer in the effects of the immediate and progressive shifts of Bennett movements (Fig. 35–1), I strongly suggest pantographing each case to determine if extreme Bennett movements are present. If we find that the patient has very little or no visible Bennett shift, we proceed in the manner described in previous chapters.

However, if there is a definite Bennett shift, if you do not incorporate it into the occlusion you will probably have continual trouble with your case.

1. Take preliminary alginate impressions (upper and lower) in the usual manner.

2. Take wash impressions using Vacustatic with either EX-3-N material or a rubber base.

3. Establish on reinforced bite blocks in the patient's mouth vertical and tentative centric occlusion through the act of swallowing, first eliminating muscle spasms.

4. Take a face bow record using the Whip Mix quick-mount face bow in order to better accommodate the next steps to the patient's skull landmarks.

5. Articulate the swallowed-in bite blocks on the Whip Mix articulator.

6. Select the position of the upper and lower anterior teeth by using Pound's method of esthetics and phonetics.

7. Select mold and color of the teeth.

8. Set up the 6 upper and lower teeth according to Steps 6 and 7 above.

9. Make a tongue index recording in order to more accurately determine the occlusal plane and, of special importance, to ascertain where to set the posterior teeth.

10. Using the tongue index, complete the upper and lower posterior portions of the set-up by using the 30° Pilkington-Turner teeth (Dentists' Supply Co.).

11. Remove these wax set-ups from the articulator and set them aside for future use during the procedure.

At this stage, we are able to go ahead with a method that has proved worth the effort in comfort and efficiency to the patient, although it requires considerable sophistication to use efficiently.

12. Employing the previously established vertical opening from the Whip Mix articulator, construct upper and lower clutches using the regular or modified[1] Denar clutches made for edentulous mouths (Fig. 35–2) according to the manufacturer's procedure manual (Fig. 35–3). At this juncture the central bearing screw is opened about 2 to 3 mm. to allow for tissue resiliency.

13. These clutches (Fig. 35–4) are now removed from the Whip Mix articulator and inserted into the mouth. Test for noninterference in centric and eccentric position by having the patient practice slid-

[1] Modification by Victor Baptist, 85 Leeuwarden Road, Darien, Connecticut, 06820

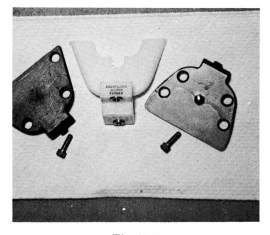

Fig. 35-2

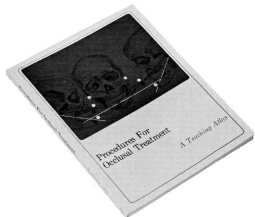

Fig. 35-3

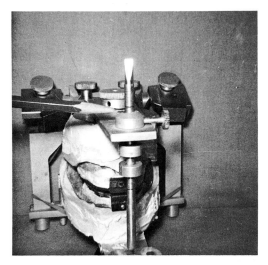

Fig. 35-4

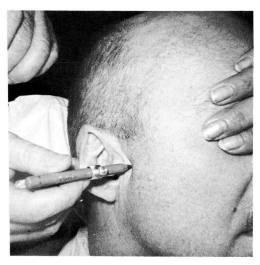

Fig. 35-5

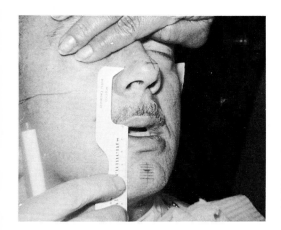

Fig. 35-6

ing these clutches on the central bearing point—forward, back and laterally.

14. Continuing to follow the procedure manual, use an arbitrary hinge axis by locating, first, posterior reference points, (Fig. 35-5) and then an anterior reference point (Fig. 35-6). (In full denture prosthesis, due to the resiliency of the ridge areas, an accurate hinge axis mounting may not be possible; if not, an arbitrary hinge axis is sufficient. However, there are those who will prefer to spend the additional time required to locate the true hinge axis.)

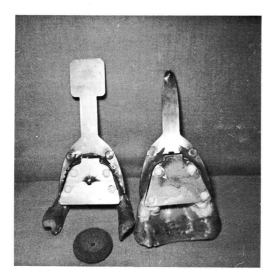

Fig. 35–7

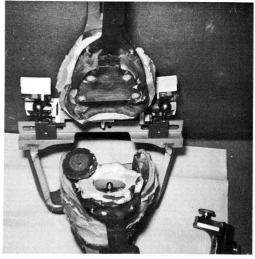

Fig. 35–8

15. Attach and assemble the pantograph to these clutches in the patient's mouth.

16. Have the patient again practice the "dry run" of sliding the mandible back and forth and laterally on the central bearing screw, making sure that there are no interferences or trippings during these movements. (The jaws must be held closed during all these movements.)

17. Activate the instrument and have the patient execute the various pantographic recordings.

18. After insuring that the centric pins are correctly locked in the wax wells, inject an anterior fast-set stone index, which acts as an additional stabilizer for the pantograph. Ascertain that the anterior reference plane locator is in place, and remove the entire attached apparatus (clutches and pantograph) from the mouth.

19. Continuing to follow the procedure manual, this entire attached apparatus is secured to the Denar D4A articulator and the upper model attached to the articulator.

20. The instrument is now programmed to the recordings registered by the pantograph, and all these recordings noted on a special form for future use.

21. Disassemble the pantograph from the clutches. If the modified Denar clutches were used, as we strongly advise, interpose a semisoft rubber-type tire. (I added a special extra-oral device[1] (Fig. 35–7), to these clutches for the recording of centric.[2]) A special ink[3] is painted on the recording table of the extra-oral device. This helps to give a distinct gothic arch tracing.

22. Take these check bite apparatuses back to the mouth and after a dry run place the rubber tire over the central bear-

[1] Obtained from Victor Baptist.
[2] This extra-oral apparatus was used because it enables you to see when the patient scribes a gothic arch tracing. While he holds on the apex, lock this position in place by means of a fast-set stone. In order to equalize the pressures on the ridges, and to assure that the intra-oral bearing is placed in the center of tissue resistance, employ a sponge rubber-type tire while the patient records the gothic tracing. Holding the patient on the apex of the gothic arch with this sponge tire interposed between the clutches and over the central bearing screw, inject fast-setting stone between the clutches. When the stone has set, the entire apparatus is removed from the mouth.
[3] Dykem Ink Co., 2307 North 11th St., St. Louis, Mo.

ing screw. Have the patient execute a gothic arch tracing.

23. While holding the patient on the apex of the gothic arch tracing, inject fast-set stone all the way around and between the upper and lower bite block clutches.

24. Remove the apparatus from the mouth when the stone has set.

25. Removed the sponge rubber tire (to enable the positioning of the stone check bite)[3] (Fig. 35–8) and place this centric stone check bite apparatus on the upper model. The lower cast is positioned into the lower clutch and the articulation completed on the Denar instrument by means of stone composition (Fig. 35–9).

26. To recheck centric occlusion, remove these clutches from the articulator, and repaint the lower platform. Then have the patient execute another gothic arch tracing, which is secured by interposing stone as was done before.

27. When the stone has set, remove the apparatus from the mouth and reinsert into the Denar articulator.

28. The centric results should be identical.

29. Remove the check bite apparatus, insert into this articulation the previously made upper and lower wax try-in set-ups and balance the occlusion to the previously programmed instrument.

30. After characterizing the buccal, lingual and palatal portions of these try-in dentures by means of Surgident flange wax, send them to the laboratory for processing.

31. Although my centric on these wax

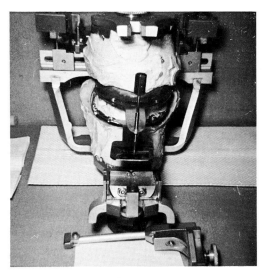

Fig. 35–9

cases check-out exactly before processing, I found after processing that a slight deviation in centric sometimes existed, but within adjustable limits.

32. This slight deviation proved how important a remount procedure is. Variations in the materials used and possibly a rotational change in the temporomandibular joint were responsible for these discrepancies. However, as long as you are aware of these changes and their contributive effect, and are able to correct them, you have recognized an important factor in building comfortable, functional dentures.

ALTERNATIVE METHOD OF ADJUSTING THE DENAR ARTICULATOR

Downward Displacement. When the stylus appears to be below the rotating condyle line on the posterior vertical recording table, it indicates a downward displacement. Remembering that the recording table moves with the mandible, it is simple to visualize that in order for the line to have been scribed the table must have been at a lower level. If no compensating adjustment is made on the superior fossa wall and the denture teeth are set in cross-arch balanced occlusion, the case exhibits disocclusion on the working side when transferred to the mouth. To compensate for this in the mouth it would be necessary to increase the progressive side shift adjustment, which has the effect of allowing for a steeper cusp height buccolingually.

Upward Displacement. When the stylus appears to be above the rotating condyle line while setting to the pantographic tracing, it indicates an upward displacement of the rotating condyle. If no compensation is made on the control surfaces of the articulator, the case will exhibit cuspal collision when transferred to the mouth. To compensate for this in the mouth and to aid in efficiently fabricating the occlusion on the articulator, it would be necessary to increase the amount of progressive side shift, which would have the effect of decreasing the cusp height buccolingually.

Posterior Displacement. When the stylus appears to be posterior to either the medial leg of the anterior gothic arch tracing on the rotating condyle side, or appears to be posterior to the rotating condyle line on the posterior horizontal recording table, it indicates posterior displacement. If this action is not compensated for in the articulator and the case is later transferred to the mouth, it exhibits cuspal collision between the distal surfaces of the lower cusps and the mesial surfaces of the upper cusps. To allow for the articulator to compensate for this movement automatically it is necessary to position the vertical axis of rotation more medially, which has a similar effect on the occlusion as a posterior displacement.

Anterior Displacement. When the stylus appears to be anterior to the medial leg of the anterior gothic arch tracing or anterior to the rotating condyle line on the posterior horizontal recording table, it indicates an anterior displacement of the rotating condyle. If this movement is not compensated for in the articulator, the case will exhibit cuspal collision between the mesial surfaces of the lower cusps and the distal surfaces of the upper cusps. To efficiently compensate for this action on the articulator it would be necessary to move the vertical axis of rotation to a more lateral position.

Bibliography

1. CONSULTATION WITH THE PATIENT AND EVALUATION OF DENTURE PROBLEMS

Brewer, A. A.: Treating complete denture patients. J. Pros. Dent. *14*: 1015, 1964.

Pound, E.: Preparatory dentures: a protective philosophy. J. Pros. Dent. *15*: 5, 1965.

LaVere, A. M.: Denture education for edentulous patients. J. Pros. Dent. *16*: 451, 1966.

4. WASH IMPRESSIONS

Kubalek, M. V., and Buffington, B. C.: Impressions by the use of subatmospheric pressure. J. Pros. Dent. *16*: 213, 1966.

7. DETERMINATION OF CORRECT ANTERIOR LENGTH AND THE PLACEMENT OF THE POST-DAM IN THE UPPER BITE BLOCK

Silverman, M. M.: Occlusion in Prosthodontics and in the Natural Dentition. Washington D.C., Mutual Publishing Co., 1962.

9. THE RECORDING OF VERTICAL AND PRELIMINARY CENTRIC RELATION THROUGH THE ACT OF SWALLOWING

Martone, A. L.: The phenomenon of function in complete denture prosthodontics. Clinical applications of concepts of functional anatomy and speech science to complete denture prosthodontics. J. Pros. Dent. *13*: 4, 204, 1963.

10. SHAPING THE UPPER BITE BLOCK AS AN AID IN SETTING THE UPPER SIX ANTERIOR TEETH

Lammie, G. A.: The position of the anterior teeth in complete dentures. J. Pros. Dent. *9*: 584, 1959.

Krajicek, D. D.: Providing a natural appearance for edentulous patients of long standing. J. Canada Dent. Assn. *33*: 502, 1967.

Silverman, M. M.: Occlusion in Prosthodontics and in Natural Dentition. Washington, D.C., Mutual Publishing Co., 1962.

11. SELECTION AND SETTING OF ANTERIOR TEETH

Lammie, G. A.: The position of the anterior teeth in complete dentures. J. Pros. Dent. *9*: 584, 1959.

Silverman, M. M.: Occlusion in Prothodontics and in Natural Dentition. Washington, D.C., Mutual Publishing Co., 1962.

12. ESTHETICS AND PHONETICS; DETERMINING THE POSITION OF THE LOWER POSTERIOR TEETH

Silverman, M. M.: The whistle and swish sound in denture patients. J. Pros. Dent. *17:* 144, 1967.

Krajicek, D. D.: Dental art in prosthodontics. J. Pros. Dent. *21:* 122, 1969.

Silverman, M. M.: Occlusion in Prosthodontics and in the Natural Dentition. Washington, D.C., Mutual Publishing Co., 1962.

13. MECHANICAL AIDS IN THE RECORDING OF CENTRIC AND ECCENTRIC POSITIONS

Michman, J., and Langer, A.: Comparison of three methods of registering centric relation for edentulous patients. J. Pros. Dent. *13*: 1066, 1964.

Buffington, B. C.: Stabilizing record bases with controlled subatmospheric pressure. J. Pros. Dent. *21*: 14, 1969.

14. RECORDING CENTRIC OCCLUSION, BENNETT MOVEMENTS AND CONDYLAR INCLINATIONS UNDER AIR-CENTRIC GOTHIC ARCH TRACINGS

Kane, B. E., and Thompson, W. C.: Improved buoyant stress equalizer. J. Pros. Dent. *17:* 365, 1967.

15. SETTING BENNETT MOVEMENTS AND CONDYLAR INCLINATIONS ON THE WHIP MIX ARTICULATOR

Cohen, R.: More on the Bennett movement. J. Pros. Dent. *9:* 388, 1959.

16. POSITIONING AND SETTING OF POSTERIOR TEETH

Friedman, S.: Principles of setups in complete dentures. J. Pros. Dent. *22:* 111, 1969.

17. RECHECKING CENTRIC OCCLUSION ON THE TRY-IN DENTURE

Berg, T., Jr., Chase, W. W., and Ray, K.: Denture base pressure tests. J. Pros. Dent. *17:* 540, 1967.

Kane, B. E., and Thompson W. C.: Improved buoyant stress equalizer. J. Pros. Dent. *17:* 365, 1967.

18. PROVIDING FOR BENNETT MOVEMENT AND CONDYLAR INCLINATIONS ON THE SET-UP

Cohen, R.: More on the Bennett Movement. J. Pros. Dent. *9:* 788, 1959.

19. CHARACTERIZATION OF THE BUCCAL, LINGUAL AND PALATAL ASPECTS OF WAX TRY-INS

Lott, F., and Levin, B.: Flange technique; and anatomic and physiologic approach to increased retention, function comfort and appearance of dentures. J. Pros. Dent. *16:* 394, 1966.

Brill, N.: Factors in the mechanism of full denture retention—discussion of selected papers. Dent. Pract., *18:* 9, 1967.

20. RECORD OF FACE BOW TRANSFER

Christiansen, R. L.: Rationale of the face-bow in maxillary cast mounting. J. Pros. Dent. *9:* 388, 1959.

21. REMOVAL OF DENTURES FROM THE ARTICULATOR AND THEIR DISPATCH TO THE LABORATORY

Peyton, F. A., and Anthony, D. H.: Evaluation of dentures processed by different techniques. J. Pros. Dent. *13:* 269, 1963.

Index